DETOUR
AGENT ORANGE

Cover photo courtesy of Shutterstock.com

Interior and cover format by Debora Lewis
arenapublishing.org

ISBN-13: 978-1719141840
ISBN-10: 1719141843

DETOUR
AGENT ORANGE

A Marine Vietnam Veteran's Battle with Total Paralysis from Guillain-Barre Syndrome Caused by Agent Orange – and His Journey Through the American Medical System

Dale M. Herder & Sam Smith

Contents

Preface

The Four Horsemen of the Apocalypse were: Pestilence, War, Famine and Death. Agent Orange could have been one of the horsemen, except for the thundering hoofs, since it approached its victims silently. But it proved to be just as devastating.

On January 27, 1973, the Vietnam War ended for the American soldiers with the Paris Peace Accord, two and a half years before the fall of South Vietnam to the communists from the north. But many American soldiers would fight another war upon returning home; they would fight the effects of Agent Orange for the rest of their lives. Guillain-Barre Syndrome is one of the diseases caused by Agent Orange.

This is the story of the detour my life took when I was ravaged by the effects of Agent Orange after serving my country.

Chapter I

Onset

They were laughing at me. I must have been staggering.

The two women coming out the door of the hospital responded to my "good morning" with nods, then one smirked as she passed me and in a low voice whispered to her friend, "He's drunk, and it isn't even noon yet."

After getting out of my car in the hospital parking lot, I had walked toward the hospital in hopes that a neurologist could tell me what was happening. The women had noted my staggered gait and heard something in my slurred speech that I wanted to deny: My body was taking an unscheduled detour from normal functioning to paralysis. I was losing control of my muscles and my body.

Thirty-five minutes before, I had left the office of my family doctor after he had spent two hours poking, prodding and puzzling. With a worried look, he said he was unable to diagnose the problem, and that he made an immediate appointment for me with a neurologist at the nearest town. When asked by his nurse if I was able to drive myself to the doctor's office, I said, "Sure, I'm fine."

I still didn't believe anything was seriously wrong. The numbness in my feet and fingers was getting worse, and my speech and swallowing were getting much harder. But the changes were gradual, almost imperceptible to me. I was sure I still could drive. After all, these were just temporary problems that would go away when the doctor diagnosed my difficulty and prescribed a pill.

The drive to the hospital would become a challenge of weakening muscles and my ability to compensate for them. To steer I locked my elbows, then I could use my shoulder muscles along with my arm muscles to steer the car. As my ability to grip the steering wheel was weakening, I used the friction of my palm against the leather covered steering wheel to turn the steering wheel. Thank goodness for power steering. I experimented with locking my elbows as I drove by trying to stay in my lane. I used cruise control to maintain a steady speed (luckily most of the drive was expressway, so no changing speeds and few curves). I rested my neck muscles by leaning back on the seat for support. As I drove toward the neurologist, the day was sunny, but storm clouds were forming for my future.

All of this had begun at 5:30 a.m., when my alarm clock went off. The date was December 16, 1981.

I was in my country home with my 11-year-old daughter, Carrie, whose custody had been awarded to me by the court after my wife and I had divorced about five years before. Our blue Great Dane, Lady, was both friend and protector of Carrie. We were a happy threesome in our home nestled on the edge of a national forest. The snow outside was a foot deep and unblemished, and the silence of the brittle cold hung over the hardwood trees that surrounded our home on the fifteen acres of woodland.

Because of my time as a Marine in Vietnam and the scorn that came with it, our simple home and fifteen acres on a river were a dream come true. I had spotted the house while driving through the countryside five years earlier. Coming around a bend in the road, I saw the house and its surroundings, and I instantly was drawn to the quiet life promised by such a place. As I drove closer, a For Sale sign said," here is a place to hide in plain sight" to a young man whose actual homecoming from combat had been anything but welcoming by the anti-Viet Nam War faction of my fellow citizens. I wanted only peace and quiet for Carrie and me after having had neither for such a very long time.

It didn't take long to obtain a VA loan so I could buy the house for Carrie, Lady, and me. And what a home it became. In the spring, blossoms perfumed the air from the six apple trees that shaded and provided more apples than we could eat. Flowers popped up to color the yard and the garden was rototilled, fertilized and planted to provide fresh vegetables in the fall. In the summer wild blackberries grew in the field next to the house, and the woods around our home were alive with the singing of all varieties of birds. A possum would harass Lady by wandering into the driveway, then play dead when Lady came bounding up. Then quietly moving on after Lady's attention turned to something else. A giant oak tree with a homemade swing for Carrie stood beside the driveway. In the fall, Carrie and I would stand in our living room watching a herd of deer that had gathered outside our window for an apple feast. As the forest around us was full of color from the leaves on the trees, the bucks, does and fawns silently grazed on the apples, and when they had their fill, quietly slipped back into the forest. The garden produced fresh vegetables in the late summer and Fall; the best was corn-on-the-cob, picked and immediately boiled. The sweetness and flavor of the corn was much greater than store bought. Fresh eggs from the hens that roamed the yard and reduced the bug population, were always available. Wild wintergreen berries and peppermint leaves grew at the edge of the forest along with mushrooms to provide tasty treats. The winter provided a rest from all the outdoor work.

We truly were blessed, hiding in plain sight, as we came to understand country living. I had found it:

A real home in which to raise my daughter and spend the rest of my life. Or so I thought.

Every morning, after shutting off the alarm clock next to my bed, I rose to get firewood for the wood-burning pot-bellied stove in our living room that heated our house all winter long. In summer and fall I was outdoors cutting fallen trees into one-foot round sections with my chainsaw. Then the round logs were split with an axe to fit into the wood stove and then neatly stacked by the back door, until I had cut plenty of wood to supply our winter warmth. But this morning, as I made my way to the pile of hardwood that I kept stacked next to the back door, I noticed something odd. My hands and feet felt numb, the same feeling I had had years ago, but then it was dismissed by corpsmen as nothing. I pressed on in my habitual morning march to stack chunks of hardwood into the crook of my left arm. Something was wrong, but it didn't register. Maybe I was just tired?

Instead of two trips to fill the wood stove, I made four. Each load seemed to feel heavier than the last, but my brain wasn't yet processing the fact that I was losing strength in both arms. It was too early in the morning to analyze what was happening to me. I needed to load the wood on top of the hot coals in the old pot-bellied stove, remnants of last night's warmth, in order to keep the house warm until I came home from work in the afternoon. And I needed to get Carrie up, get her ready for school, and get myself ready for work.

The red coals left over from the previous night fire, were perfect to ignite my armloads of aged oak logs as I fed, piece after piece, the new day's fire. I had gotten the wood stove at a second-hand store in the nearby town in which my three older siblings and I had been raised with no mother – and an absent father. I had built a slave brick base and wall behind the wood stove to absorb the heat and radiate it back out evenly. The multicolor brick gave the stove a quaint look. On the brick base I would stack the wood before I loaded the stove. The kitchen table was an antique hardwood, circular with an ornamental base. In the living room I had built a plant holder, which was filled with easy care plants to brighten the winter days. The living room walls were Knotty Pine that I had cut and nailed to the walls. The living room had a large picture window. The furniture was functional, some antique, some second hand. The look was not the tie-dye bright and colorful that was popular, but simple and muted.

By 7 a.m. I had had two cups of coffee, and the chill was gone from our home. I awakened Carrie, and after she had washed up and tumbled into her school clothes I told her that I planned to stay home and go to the doctor. She said, "Daddy, I'll stay home, too, and make you some soup." Her offer was not the typical manipulative technique of an eleven-year-old. She could see that I was worried.

I thanked her, gave her a hug, and nudged her out the door toward the flashing lights of the yellow school bus that had just stopped on our country road at the edge of our driveway. The driver waved, got Carrie settled into a seat, and motored down the road to our neighbor's house. As I waved to Carrie, little did I know that I also was waving goodbye to my life style that I had slowly built.

By the time Carrie sat down in the bus, my hands and feet were deeply numb. It felt as if they were being stuck by a thousand needles. Reality of the seriousness of my condition began to sink in with the pierce of each needle.

Was I in denial? What the Hell was going on?

I realized that I had lost my manual dexterity when I couldn't use my finger to operate our rotary-dial wall phone to call my sister. It was important to let someone know that there was a problem, so I improvised, I wedged a pencil between my fingers and clumsily was able to dial the number of my sister, Linda. I told her about my numbness, how weak I felt, and that I was planning to call my local doctor when his office opened in an hour. As she talked, Linda tried to reassure me, but her words seemed hollow as my body was telling me something my brain wouldn't accept.

My instincts were clicking into gear as they had many times before in a distant and foreign land, and, just as then, I sensed that this situation could go bad fast.

After more than two hours of probing, my local doctor's opinion was simple and direct: My reflexes were gone, and the rest of my muscle nerves were failing as well. But why? He didn't know, so he called the neurologist whose office in the next town was at the other end of the hospital parking lot where the two women were to tsk-tsk me for being a staggering drunk before noon.

As the women coming out of the hospital sneered at me, my awkward gait became almost a stumble and my eyes began to lose focus. Somehow I was able to squint and find the doctor's name on the wall directory to find the office number.

The doctor's receptionist said she expected me, and she immediately ushered me into a patient examination room to wait for the doctor. "Please sit down," she said.

That was it.

I would never walk again.

The neurologist came into the room. Like a professional he conducted electric shock tests on my hands, arms, legs, and feet. He was trying to find something that would give him a clue as to what was happening to me. The electrical current should have caused my muscles to jerk, to react... to do something. Instead... nothing. Not a damned thing, just the pain from the electrical shocks.

I was going numb, but my pain sensation still was working. I still felt all the pokes and stabs from the doctor's instruments though the numbness. After an hour of testing, probing, and flat and unresponsive hits on my elbows and knees with a small rubber hammer, the evidence was clear. My nerves were not conducting the message to my muscles to make them work. But the neurologist couldn't tell me why, exactly.

I was an electrician. That meant I was a trouble-shooter, then fix-it man. Every day was for me, a process of elimination. Test it. Analyze it. Start with the most probable cause of the problem. If that was not the problem, move on to the next possible cause. Find the problem and then fix it. Why wasn't the doctor doing this?

I wanted, needed, answers.

My world was spinning out of control. I was losing the ability to control my muscles, and, as I was to find out the hard way, when we have no control of our bodies we have no control of the world around us. My mind began to shift from analysis to damage control, and my emotions skidded from quiet dread to managed panic.

In the end a wheelchair was bought into the room to move me into the hospital. With the limited strength I had left, I was able to slide from the doctor's examining table to the wheelchair, and the doctor ordered my immediate admission to the Intensive Care Unit to further evaluate me and find the cause of what was happening to me.

"The Intensive Care Unit? What is happening to me?" I asked him.

He offered no answer, but when he turned away it was with a look on his face that said things I didn't want to hear. Even with all his medical training and experience, he had no idea what was happening to me.

In my own mind I thought: "This must be a mistake; I'm way too healthy to be in a hospital, let alone ICU."

As I was being pushed out of the office toward Intensive Care, I asked the receptionist to call my sister. I mumbled the telephone number. Linda needed to be told that I was being admitted. She needed to take care of Carrie.

Chapter II

The Terror

They say the road to Hell is paved with good intentions. My road to Hell was paved with indifference.

It started with the first person I met on my way to ICU... a hospital admission clerk.

The Marine Corps taught me not to bellyache, and I don't ask for much from anyone. But the cold, uncompassionate order, "Give me the name of your insurance company," didn't match what was happening to me. My mind was spinning, trying to process the events of this morning. I could do little more than mumble a response. My tongue felt too thick to fit in my mouth. The tone of her voice didn't have any compassion that it should have had when talking to a patient about to enter ICU. I was in serious trouble and she was someone who didn't care. She seemed more interested in getting the form filled out, so she could return to her crossword puzzle or computer solitaire game.

I needed to know who would care for my daughter and what in the hell was happening to me. The cold, robotic clerk behind the desk expressed no interest in me or my rapidly deteriorating condition. She understood nor saw nothing about the person she was talking to. All she cared about was the paperwork she needed to fill out. I struggled to control my vocal cords and tongue in order to speak, and after the clerk typed the name of my health insurance company, she asked, in the same dull monotone, "If you die, who do we notify?" I stared at her in disbelief. She sounded as if she were ordering salami on rye.

Dante described the fires of Hell in *The Inferno*. Dante was the same age as I, when he started his journey to Hell. He was greeted by the sign *"Abandon all hope, ye who enter here."* I must have missed seeing that sign as I left the doctor's office and entered into the hospital. I was spiraling downward into what I would later come to understand as the Hell of Guillain-Barre Syndrome, a neurological disease that would hit me as hard as it has ever hit anyone who survived it. As I was talking to the admissions clerk, it was ripping the myelin sheath from my nerves, making my muscles useless. Although I didn't know it then, Guillain-Barre would take me more than once to Hell's door. But right now Hell's door was being held open by the hospital clerk with the expressionless face and empty eyes, who was filling out the entrance hospital form.

I was becoming a 35-year-old, 6-foot 4-inch, 220-pound slab of meat... with a fully functioning brain and a non-functional body with no way to express my thought or feelings.

Within twenty-four hours I would lose all control of my body, and most of my humanity went with it.

After my interrogation by the admissions clerk, an orderly wheeled me to a bed in ICU. He dropped the side rail and motioned for me to get into the bed. With what little strength I had left, and unable to fully stand up, I dragged myself from the wheel chair into the bed. Just sheer willpower kept me from collapsing onto the floor. My fingers were no longer functioning, so a nurse had to help undress me and put on what I was to wear for the next thirteen months – a hospital gown. My hospital room cost more per day than the best rooms in the finest hotels, so I expected to be treated at least with courtesy and respect while the medical team sorted out what was happening to me.

Quite the contrary.

No one asked how I was feeling. No one said, "Excuse me for making you naked." No one asked, "Are you comfortable?" Simple courtesies ended when I became 100% paralyzed and totally vulnerable.

No one said or asked anything, and the silence was deafening. Was the indifference a result of fear on the part of the staff, or was it the result of inadequate training and low standards at a small-town hospital?

My vulnerability led to a ghostly invisibility. No one on the hospital staff seemed to know that I was there. If anyone peeked into my room, he or she apparently saw only a bed. Then it hit me: Maybe... just maybe... no one really cared.

Later that night, when I had to urinate and could not get out of bed to get to the bathroom, a nurse simply came into my room and dropped a urinal into which I was to pee, and said press the call button to tell her I was done. She turned and left the room without a word. She had no idea of the condition of her patient. No longer possessing manual dexterity, I discovered that moving the hospital gown aside was a formidable task, as part of it was underneath me. By now I lacked the muscles to sit up. Rolling to one side to move the hospital gown out from under me, so I could move it to one side to place the urinal under the gown, was hard. The use of the fingers to grab the gown and move it was gone. Holding the urinal in place was impossible. And, like most of us, I had never learned how to pee while lying down. The predictable result was a badly wet bed.

When the nurse came back, she was upset that the bed had to be changed. She was more concerned about having to do work than the fact that a patient was in distress and humiliated. I tried to mumble my apology and shame, but nothing came out.

Strangely, as I lay in the ICU bed I wasn't conscious of the slow paralysis of my body, and I wasn't especially conscious of the fact that the energy was slowly draining from my body. Exhaustion from trying to do simple things, like rolling over, seeped through me slowly, imperceptibly, as numbness took its toll.

I had nothing to read and was unable to work the remote, so I could not watch television. As a result, I was unable to notice that my eye muscles were weakening, that my eyes were not focusing normally. My temperature and heart rate would become wildly erratic as my nervous system deteriorated.

As the night wore on I had too much time to think. I had never been in a hospital as a patient. All of this was new, confusion filled my thoughts, as in my mind I replayed the day. What had happened to get me here? But surely the doctors would sort this mess out... wouldn't they? They think logically like an electrician, use a simple process of elimination, write things down, try new things, find the cause, and fix it... don't they?

Maybe I was in shock. Things happening to my body were happening very fast, and I had never experienced a serious illness, so I had nothing with which to compare to this demon. Little did I know that my world already had changed forever.

Somehow, as I lay in that ICU bed that evening, I had the impression that I would wake up in the morning just as I had been when I had gone to bed the night before – healthy and ready to raise my daughter, do my job, pay the bills. I had worked with my hands since I had turned eighteen years old. I needed my paycheck every week.

Never in my life had I enjoyed social or financial privileges. So, if I didn't work, I wouldn't get paid. That's how the world works, doesn't it? No work, no pay?

There were bills on the kitchen table that would be overdue in two weeks. My daughter was only 11 years old. I was a single dad with serious responsibilities. I had no time, no patience, for this sickness.

The neurologist's receptionist made the call to my sister, Linda, at the redi-mix concrete business she and her husband owned. Once Linda realized that I was being hospitalized, she called Carrie's maternal aunt and asked her to pick Carrie up after school. The aunt had her husband pick up Carrie. Linda also called my other sister, Diane, at her law office.

Aunt Sandy called Carrie at home after school, where Carrie was watching an afternoon TV educational special with Lady at her side. Carrie, just off the school bus, was unaware of my situation or that I was in the Intensive Care Unit. Aunt Sandy took charge: "Pack your suitcase, Carrie.

Your daddy is in the hospital, and I will send my husband to come and get you so you can stay at our house."

Knowing no details, and having no choice other than to trust the adults in her world, my 11-year-old girl packed her red plastic suitcase with its red plastic handle. Her uncle arrived, loaded Carrie into the car, locked Lady in the house, and moved my daughter to her temporary home. I will always regret the loss of a friend, my Great Dane, Lady. She was a member of the family and I was helpless to protect her from her fate. Lady would eventually be given away and probably never understood what had happened to her family.

After two nights at Aunt Sandy's home, Carrie was moved to her grandmother's home. Her grandmother was a nice lady, who often babysat for her. So, it was a better place for my daughter to be. She was picked up a few days later by her Uncle Don, who had driven down from his cement plant with his two daughters, Denise and Sandy. By that time, Don had become a harried temporary bachelor. Linda and Diane, my two sisters, already were in town to be with me at the hospital, and Don was ill-prepared to be the solo husband in charge of his two daughters and a redi-mix cement plant business. To make things even more "interesting" for Don, he and Linda had agreed to move Carrie into their daughters' room and enroll her in elementary school for the second half of sixth grade. Don would have three girls to supervise—and no wife to run the front office at the cement plant. All of this just when the cement business finally was getting on its financial feet after six years of constant struggle to make a profit.

My sisters are organizers. As soon as they had gotten off the phone with each other, they began to plan how they could free up things in their lives in order to come to the hospital.

Linda began to plan how she could get away from her cement plant desk in the next few days, if needed, and Diane cleared her teaching and law office desks, made plans to drive the hundred miles to my bedside immediately, and called her husband, Dale, at his office. My brother-in-law called his father, who lived in the same town as the hospital I was in and asked him to go across the city so I would have someone at my side in ICU. He told his father that I must be in serious condition to be placed in ICU.

Less than one hour after making her phone calls, Diane loaded her sons into their car and set off for the long drive to the hospital on a wintry and icy night.

As I lay in the hospital bed alone and wondering what was happening, Dale's father arrived at the hospital. I didn't know it at the time, but he would be one of the last persons, I would be able to speak with for many months to come. I struggled to get out the few words, because of shortness of breath. I asked if my daughter was being taken care of. If my message had gotten through to my sister. Dale's dad told me that my message to my sisters had been received, and that Carrie was safe and being watched over by a relative. Seemed like the first time since being admitted, someone was treating me as though I was human. He stayed for an hour or so until my sister arrived.

When Diane arrived at the hospital it was dark. She talked to her father-in-law, then the hospital staff. Then she sent her sons home with her father-in-law as she prepared to spend as much of the night with me in the ICU, as the hospital staff would let her.

As the night grew late, Diane and I talked about what was happening to me and how my sickness had come on. She asked questions of the hospital staff, and she began to take notes. Maybe it was her law training. Maybe it was her training as a Soviet historian. Whatever the reason, she began to write down whatever she could learn and pass on to the next family member who would arrive. One nurse upon seeing the notes, said, "You guys just keep taking notes."

Did that nurse know something we didn't yet know?

I was totally paralyzed by the time my other sister, Linda, arrived the following day and looked through the notes that Diane had given to her when she got to my bedside. By then, I could move nothing but my eyes.

I listened as Linda asked the nurse in my room about my medical status. The nurse said, "There is nothing you can do. He's in a coma. He doesn't understand anything that is going on around him, he doesn't feel anything, and he doesn't hear anything."

I will never forget hearing the nurse's words. I couldn't move, but in my mind I was screaming: "You are wrong. You are wrong. I am here. I can hear you. I am not in a coma. Look at me and see that I'm conscious."

But my sister and the nurse heard nothing and saw no movement. There was nothing I could do that would suggest to them that I was conscious, listening to every word that was spoken about me.

I felt a shadow pass over me as I heard the nurse's words. The shadow of a casket lid closing just above my face. Suddenly my hospital bed had become my coffin. Death wore a nurse's uniform, and it was her hand that was guiding the closing lid.

The nurse's words would be worse than any death sentence I could receive. No one would know that I was alive and alert. I could hear Death laughing in my mind and could see that its bony skeleton hand was closing the coffin lid. I could feel the silky casket lid inches from my face. Trapped with no one knowing I was still alive. No one to hear me screaming in my mind, no one to see me mentally clawing at the lid....

Then remarkably, I heard my sister say, "Sam, if you understand me, blink three times." With Death masquerading as the nurse who still was at my bedside, I felt the casket lid starting to leave death's control and a struggle begin to raise the lid.

I probably blinked fifteen times. It wasn't clear to me that Linda saw in my eyes that I was conscious, but thank God she was asking me to communicate.

She hesitated, and then I knew... I knew... that she had seen my eye blinks and understood that I was alert, able to hear, able to respond.

The nurse didn't believe that I was communicating in response to Linda's prompt. She said, "Those blinks are just a reflex reaction; he's not really conscious."

So Linda said, "Do it again, Sam. Blink three times."

I blinked precisely three times, not wanting to give the nurse anything to doubt. I was fighting to maintain control and blinked once, twice, three times, then stopped and waited for their reaction.

Not another blink.

The nurse turned on her heel and left the room. Death temporarily stepped back into the shadows of my room to watch and await its next move.

It knew.

The close encounter with Death triggered a memory from Viet Nam, where I had served in the infantry as a Marine fire team leader in charge of four Marines:

We were moving through the countryside by a village; it might have appeared to be a show of force (if twelve Marines were a "force"). But in reality we were looking the area over for a good ambush site for the coming night. We were there to protect the villagers. The North Vietnamese would sneak into the villages at night to "intimidate" the villagers. The intimidation consisted of stealing food, killing village leaders, who didn't agree with them, and raping women. When we returned home after a thirteen-month tour in Viet Nam, we were met by a public that portrayed us as baby killers, cowards and drug addicts. Yet, I still remember an old villager giving us Kool-Aid to drink after one hard-fought night outside his village. As we passed through his village in the morning, he came out and offered us a drink and a slight bow. Although it was a simple act of gratitude for putting our lives at risk to defend strangers, it said more to me than any Oliver Stone movie ever could. And the media reported none of these atrocities committed by the North Vietnamese.

We had selected an ambush site outside the village in a cemetery on the path that led to the village, as we moved though the countryside on patrol earlier in the day. We moved back from the patrol to our daytime position in an abandoned school house and we waited for dark before returning to the site (so as not to give away our position and the element of surprise). As our all-night vigil began at the ambush site, so did the rain. We had chosen a place where a cemetery overlooked a path to the village. On the other side of the path and lower were rice paddies that were divided into squares by dikes that were about a foot high. We were inexperienced in combat and had made elaborate plans on how the ambush would be set off. We soon would discover that the darkness, rain and the fog of combat would change our best laid plans.

The North Vietnamese walked into our ambush around midnight. Two thirds of us were sleeping (we were three Marines to a position, one was awake on watch and two sleeping, who was on watch rotated every hour). With the closeness of the enemy (less than six feet away), the rain, and two thirds of us sleeping, the plan fell apart immediately. I watched as the enemy walked into our ambush a few feet away. Knowing that moving in an effort to awaken my buddies would have eliminated the element of surprise and given the enemy the chance to shoot first and wound or *kill all of us in the first position. So, I initiated the ambush by detonating a claymore mine. Immediately the North Vietnamese began firing back, dragging their wounded and moving away from us out into the rice paddy for the protection of the dikes. I was the only Marine shooting (since two thirds of us were sleeping, they awoke disoriented and the rain and darkness was hiding the NVA from the other Marines). I was told later, by Marines stationed on a nearby ambush, that it was quite a show. My orange-red tracer bullets going out into the rice paddy and their blue-green tracer bullets coming back at me. This deadly show continued until the surviving North Vietnamese gave up the fight and escaped, leaving behind their dead.*

The grave we had chosen for our fighting position had a concrete wall round it. I was behind the wall, which was a couple of feet above the path, and the wall was only a few feet high. The rice paddy was a couple of feet below the path. The rice paddy was a crisscross of dikes. As the enemy moved off of the path and out into the rice paddy, I had to stand to see where I was shooting, and most of my body was exposed to their gunfire. It wasn't courage or bravery, just a thoughtless adaptation to the situation. As the enemy moved from dike to dike, I saw shadows of human forms that were easy to spot by the tracers coming from them. The firefight was brief but intense.

The next morning, we returned to the ambush site. The grave wall I was using for cover was pockmarked with bullet holes, just inches below where I had been standing and firing. A few inches higher and their bullets would have torn into my body. Life and death can be measured in inches.

As my mind returned from my combat memory to the hospital bed and my sister, I thought that again the difference between life and death was measured in inches, the fraction of an inch my eye lids moved as they blinked out my only way to communicate with the world outside of my mind.

I was beginning to feel as if I were a disembodied head, detached from my paralyzed body. My mind still worked. I was determined that I would not be buried alive. Linda had the presence of mind and the guts to follow her instinct, despite the intimidation of a professional nurse whose bad judgment would have marked me for a more miserable and slow death than the bullets in the graveyard half a world away.

When Diane returned to stand her watch that second day, Linda told her to talk to me. She understood that I needed to express what was happening to me and to know I wasn't isolated within my own mind. The three of us immediately began to develop an eye blink code so I could communicate.

Later that day, as I slipped further into the paralysis, I lost the ability to blink my eyes, because the nerves to my eyelid muscles were affected and the eyelids no longer worked. We discovered that I still could roll my left eye up and down and from side to side, but I needed someone to open my eyelids.

We developed an eye blink code that evolved within hours into a new eye roll code, and it was all I had to communicate with the world outside my mind for months to come.

Here is how it worked:

To get attention, I would roll my left eye up and down several times.

Once noticed, I'd be asked " Is the first letter in the first half of the alphabet?"

An upward roll of my eye meant yes. A sideways movement of my eye meant no. My family member then would recite the appropriate half of the alphabet, letter-after-letter, and an upward eye roll meant that we had arrived at the desired letter.

This continued until I spelled out the message. It was slow and tedious. But it worked, and it saved me pain and suffering more than once, as I was able to communicate problems I had with the hospital and equipment. Most important, it was my only window to the world. Try to imagine being shut in a place that you couldn't interact with things around you. Not being able to move. Not being able to speak. Not being heard. Not being able to control anything. It is like being buried alive. That was my world for the coming months, if I couldn't speak to the world outside my brain.

We developed abbreviations within our code to speed things up. "Exercise arms" became "ea," "put ice in mouth" became "im," "exercise legs" became "el," and "put ice on forehead" became "ih." Each of these shortcuts were extremely important because without the exercise to my arms and legs, the joints would freeze over time. Without being able to eat or drink, my mouth would dry and cause medical problems, the ice prevented that. The eye-rolling code was my only window to the outside world while my mind was trapped in my body for over four months.

Later, after my sisters were ordered by the nursing staff to leave my ICU room, I communicated my fears to them during the few brief visits that were allowed. Linda and Diane immediately made it clear to hospital staff that they would stay in my room at all times. The nursing staff put up a fight. The nurses said that my sisters were encouraging my paranoia by remaining in my room all the time. They insisted that Linda and Diane had to leave, period. What the staff did not understand was that I was paying for the hospital room. I think a few of them felt their authority was being challenged.

I made it clear to my sisters that I was not paranoid; rather, I was fearful for my wellbeing because of the clumsiness, unprofessional behavior and lack of caring by a few of the staff when my sisters were not in the room.

Diane, my lawyer sister, immediately went to court to get control of the situation. She filed a petition for guardianship. Based on the persuasive testimony by my sister, the judge issued an immediate writ that gave her the power of guardianship. An hour after the writ was issued, my sister presented the writ to the hospital staff. They saw with the court order, they had no choice but to allow relatives in my room, no matter what the "normal" visiting hours were. To me it was a relief and a justification of my position of needing protection. Not to mention that I was paying a hefty fee for the room and should be allowed some say in its use.

Time was not my friend. When I was left in one position too long, the weight of my body was supported on a few points that became pressure points, which if the pressure was not relieved would become painful. Further if I was left in that position long enough, the pressure points would turn into open bed sores. After twenty minutes in one position, at the pressure points I began to feel as if a lighted match was being held against my skin. Only the eye-rolling code allowed me to communicate that I was in pain and needed to be repositioned. There was no medical device to alert the staff or my family.

One major drawback of our otherwise ingenious communication system was the demand it placed on my family. They were beside my bed 24 hours a day, and they worked in solo shifts. While on watch, however, they could not sit and read a book or watch TV while I slept with my eyes open (I could not close my eyes). My "watch stander" family members had to remain high enough above my bedside to look down into my left eye, an eerie assignment, in case I rolled it up and down rapidly to tell them that I wanted to say something.

Of course, when I was sleeping with my eyes open any involuntary eye twitches when dreaming, would prompt the family member to wake me up by saying, "Sam, do you want to say something?"

Ironically, I could sleep, but my bedside family members could not sleep while on duty, no matter what hour of the night or day. No one can keep up a vigil like that. So, if they missed a call from me, I wasn't upset. I knew shortly they would see me signaling and respond.

My initial terror started to take on all the characteristics of Stalin's prisoners in the Soviet prisons. It was out of my control to be placed in this situation. I couldn't protect myself or change what was happening to me. I could only hold on tight to the shred of hope that eventually I would recover.

Chapter III

Family to the Rescue

During the first twenty-four hours of my paralysis, my family could not know what was coming, they could only helplessly watch my condition continued to deteriorate.

Their adjustments to their lifestyles went on without me being aware of it, but how they responded, and how quickly they acted, made a big difference to whether or not I would survive. Their lives and mine took a major detour when I was wheeled into the ICU. Looking back, it is now obvious that our lives came together at that point and changed direction. Like a pebble thrown into a pond, the ripples spread out from that event. Everyone's life was affected. Maybe not as earth shattering as my detour from able-bodied to quadriplegic, but at least a gentle nudge to alter the future course of the families' lives.

One of the first notes I eye-blinked from my bed in the Intensive Care Unit was, "Sorry to bother you." Taken out of context, the message might sound superficial or inconsequential. Nothing could be farther from reality.

I tend to be quiet, and I highly value self-reliance and resourcefulness. Even now as a quadriplegic, it is embarrassing for me to ask for help from anyone. Self-sufficiency is my life style, so when I blinked my "Sorry to bother you" note to the family members who were to remain at my bedside twenty-four hours a day, for three months, I meant it.

I felt as though I was spinning downward, like I was falling into the rabbit hole in Alice in Wonderland. The absurd became reality in my hospital room. Instead of having the white knight talking backwards or a red queen screaming off with her head, it was medical jargon and defense of the way the medical staff always did things. I knew that my family was key to controlling the Alice in Wonderland aspect of my care. Without the hospital staff communicating with me, I couldn't affect the care. In the end the best of the hospital staff did learn to communicate with me, the others were the red queen....

None of my family members were born with silver spoons in our mouths, and our growing-up years had more than the usual number of bumps and detours.

When the phone rang at Linda's desk at the concrete plant that she and her husband owned, she slowly absorbed the words spoken by my neurologist's receptionist. Linda jotted the details on a notepad and said, "Let Sam know that I have received this call and that we will make sure Carrie is taken care of." Her message was not relayed to me.

Linda then spoke to her husband and said, "I need to get to the hospital as soon as possible." She then made plans to leave the next morning.

As soon as Linda finished talking with her husband, she called our sister.

Diane picked up the phone at her law office and, like Linda, she went into action. Diane then was teaching English, History, and Journalism at a high school during the day, and holding the fort in the office at her solo law practice on a small town's Main Street after school and on Saturdays. She had a lot of loose ends to tie up if she was to leave in order to take advantage of the remaining daylight for the two-hour drive to my hospital.

Grabbing her pen, Diane made a to-do list for her secretary at the law office. She then made a second list to be left on the kitchen counter for her husband. Finally, she made a set of lesson plans for a substitute teacher to take over her five different high school classes for the next two days.

She called her husband to tell him the bad news. He said, "Take Roy and Dave out of school and go to the hospital. Call me tonight from the hospital to let me know if I should come over. I'll try to get approval to be gone from the office, if I am needed.

Also, I'll call my dad right away, and ask him to get to Sam's bedside right now."

Diane picked up her sons, Roy and David, got permission from her high school principal boss to be gone for the next two days, gave him her lesson plans, and left a note on the counter at home. She and the boys grabbed a change of clothes and their toothbrushes, and they were on the road by 4 p.m.

Diane felt only one emotion: Fear. Since I never had been sick or one to complain, Diane feared that my condition was serious, and she was worried how Carrie was handling the situation and how she was being cared for. As she drove, Diane tried to keep the boys occupied in the car so they would not realize how frightened she was. She did not want to scare them, and they already were confused about driving to the hospital on a school night—especially when they had to play in a hockey game two nights later.

Back in Northern Michigan, Linda put things in order overnight, packed her bags, and left home early the next morning for the 200-mile drive down Lake Michigan's coast. An hour later, at 6 a.m., she stopped at an outdoor pay phone in a gas station to call home and make sure everyone was up and getting ready for school and work. She also wanted Don and the girls, Denise and Sandy, to know she had made it half-way to the hospital on the snowy highways.

She fretted about what would happen at home. Linda knew the girls were very capable, and she said to herself, "They'll be ok; I've trained them well." Linda knew the girls would be cut off from social activities if she couldn't drive them to town and school from their rural home. But the girls seemed to understand that their mom needed to be with me at the hospital.

Once Linda arrived at the hospital, she was briefed in detail by Diane and the medical staff, and both sisters decided to stay with me to learn what was happening. It was quickly evident that my situation was spiraling out of control by the minute. By the time Linda arrived, physicians had made plans to put me on a respirator. Diane's icy-road trip with her boys the evening before had been completed in three hours, and she made arrangements on a hospital pay phone to rent a room at the Christian Home for the Aged, just a block from my hospital. She knew right away that because of my rapidly deteriorating condition, she would not be going home in the foreseeable future.

A week later, after sharing the same room and the same bed (they never saw each other at their rented room at the Christian Home, since they met only when they relieved each other and passed along their written medical notes before going at my bedside), they found a small, furnished apartment three miles from the hospital. That small apartment served as home base for my sisters for the next three months. The winter was fittingly one of the snowiest and coldest winters in recent Michigan history. Snowfall reached over fourteen feet that winter, and snow banks on the sides of streets commonly towered to fifteen or twenty feet. Temperatures circled zero for weeks during January and February as Linda and Diane drove with bright orange flags on their radio antennas so they could be seen among the snow banks and at intersections.

The only time Linda and Diane ever got to spend at the apartment together was when one of their husbands drove in to stand watch with me on weekends. Dale arrived nearly every Friday night. He stayed with me through Friday night until noon on Saturday, when he went to the apartment to sleep after being relieved at my bedside by Linda or Diane. During these once-a-week seventeen-hour respites, my sisters could do laundry, buy groceries, get eight continuous hours of sleep, and cook a casserole to be frozen for consumption later in the week, between their 12-on and 12-off watches.

Fatherhood was a theoretical and foreign term for my dad. Linda ultimately was responsible for pressuring him to pick up the rent for the apartment. For reasons unknown to me, father didn't understand, speak of, or practice love for his children.

Thus, when I became sick, my father had no idea what to do. The humming machines, IV's, wires, and tubes around my bed in the ICU overwhelmed him, and he simply was not up to spelling words out one-by-one, using our eye-roll method. He only finished fourth-grade. Education was not normal for a farm boy in the 1920s. His lack of education in spelling and arithmetic made the communication of eye-rolls with me well above his abilities and caring for a sick son was not in his emotional abilities.

Diane and Linda discussed their living situation, and Linda, being the eldest, said, "Diane, let me handle this; I'll get father to pay for the apartment."

A little background: As soon as she knew she would be staying for an extended period, Linda had asked our father to go north to her home to help Don and the girls. Her goal was to provide supervision for the children when they had to be alone in their home. When she asked for his help, father told her flatly, "no," she waited a few days. Then she said, "Dad, you weren't there when we were growing up. Few people get a second chance in life. I am giving you a second chance. Please go up and stay at our home with the girls and Don."

He said "no" again, but he agreed to pay for the apartment. He lacked the emotional family ties to step up and be a grandfather. This lack of character he carried to his grave. Even well after I left the hospital, he never tried to connect with me. I think he believed that paying the rent for his daughters was his only responsibility.

Diane and Linda settled into their 12-on and 12-off schedule at the one-bedroom apartment. The bitter cold made it difficult to keep the place warm, and they wrestled with a snow shovel every day in order to clear the icy, wooden, outdoor stairway that took them up to the second floor outdoor landing. Their shared living experience as adults became an opportunity to "camp out" like kid sisters again, but under stressful conditions that were caused by my illness and their families' needs for them to be home.

They quickly learned that they still were compatible, but very different people. They also learned that Linda's strict adherence to healthy foods was the opposite of Diane's penchant to keep M&M's with peanuts in a handy dish on the kitchen table. It was essential, Diane thought, that watch standers be able to grab a few "power pellets" (they were not candy!) on the way to and from trips to the hospital. Linda almost agreed, since getting meals at the hospital was not always possible, depending on my condition at any moment during the day or night. According to Diane's theory, a pocketful of power pellets might see a person through the last six hours of a long night watch. Chocolate, after all, helps keep a person alert. And peanuts are nutritious, aren't they?

Of my two sisters, Linda is the more theoretical, the more cautious, the more detailed, the more linear. Diane, on the other hand, is less detailed and more prone to take risks. She thinks in practical terms.

Unfortunately, Linda felt stress from home that I did not know about at the time. Her husband, Don, wanted her to be with the girls and him. In phone calls Linda made from her and Diane's apartment, Don told Linda that he and the girls needed her to return. "I wouldn't do for my parents what you are doing for your brother, and I want you to come home. If you don't, I will divorce you!"

Don eventually came to see Linda and me, and he helped at the hospital a few times. Later, after Denise and Sandy were grown, Linda and Don's marriage ended in divorce and Linda since has remarried happily.

My brother, Stan, drove up to the hospital from his home within the first two weeks of my hospitalization. Since there was a seven-year age gap between us, we never were close growing up. We didn't do things together. My illness didn't change that. There were no personal messages being passed between us. We didn't connect as brother-to-brother, despite my paralysis and continued deterioration of my health.

After five or six days, Stan bade me farewell.

Chapter IV

My Daughter Faces Changes

My hospitalization had a double-edged impact on my 11-year-old daughter. Carrie was the most frightened, youngest – and the most protected – of all my immediate family members. It was good that she was kept away from the hospital and the trauma of my worst two months in the ICU.

I wasn't pretty. I lay almost totally naked for over three months with only a folded sheet over me most of the time, for modesty, not warmth. I had tubes in nearly every orifice, and a respirator incessantly blew and sucked my chest up and down through what seemed to me to be a tailpipe-size hose stuck down a hole cut into the base of my throat. Liquid food ran into my stomach through a tube into my left nostril, and periodic doses of highly caustic potassium that were fed through the same tube caused me to wretch involuntarily and silently while I turned bright red because of the intense pain it caused as it ate away at my stomach. I asked for bananas to be crushed and fed through the feeding tube in my nose, but the doctor felt he needed to get my potassium levels up quickly, no matter what the cost. Bananas, he said, weren't good enough sources of potassium that I needed right away. I continued to wretch and turn red in intense pain before the frightened eyes of my watch standers when I was given a dose of potassium. All of this I didn't want my daughter to witness.

It was good that my sisters managed Carrie's life and kept her mind on other things as much as possible during the down side of my syndrome. At that point, we could barely hope there would be an upside to come.

Carrie's first awareness that I was sick came early on that fateful morning, when I told her I was not going to work because I was going to see a doctor. She had wanted to stay home and make soup for me—to take care of Dad, since he never missed work. I told her to get on the bus and that I would be OK. She smiled, waved, and got on the bus, as she was told.

When she got home from school that afternoon, she let herself into the house as usual, was greeted our Great Dane, Lady, as always, and settled down to watch an afternoon special children's program on TV with Lady at her side. Little did Carrie know, her life was about to detour to a new path into adulthood and femininity when she hurriedly packed her little red plastic suitcase for the drive to her Aunt Sandy's house. Packing a suitcase was a totally new business for my little girl, since we rarely took overnight trips and I was always there to help her pack the suitcase. Her overnight visits to her grandmother's house needed only PJs and a change of clothes, which did not require a suitcase.

Marine Corps crispness and neatness were not part of our routine, since the spit and polish of boot camp had been tempered by living in the field in Vietnam. Being in the infantry and combat meant sleeping on the ground in the monsoon season, with water and mud flowing over me. We would spend four days in the field, meaning no shelter or mess halls. We slept in the open, behind bushes or whatever cover we could hide behind. We only carried ammunition and food. It was impossible to carry extra clothes, besides the clothes would get wet and be heavy. We were constantly wet to the point that sores formed on my feet during monsoon season. Also, I had the red clay from Khe Sanh caked into my only set of clothes for three months, where home was a hole dug into the side of a trench line and protection from the rain when on watch was a poncho. At Khe Sanh water was scarce, so bathing was impossible. So my Vietnam experience had shown me that spit and polish was not the most important thing in life. Carrie learned from me, then I became ill. So living with my family, my daughter learned some lessons about style and femininity that I just could not teach her.

During those post-Vietnam years, my theory of parenthood revolved around something I had not had as a child... parental love. Right or wrong, I felt that Carrie needed security and unconditional love from her father, rather than starched clothing.

As Carrie and her little red suitcase rode with her Uncle Bill to spend a few nights with them, she had no idea what was happening.

After an early childhood that was deeply insecure, living with her mother in environments that were unfit for her, sleeping on the floors of different friends of her mom night after night, Carrie felt I finally had saved her by gaining custody of her young life. Now all that was in jeopardy.

By age 11 she knew that her mother had not been making good decisions, and Carrie was relieved to live in our country home in the woods, with our pot-bellied stove, Lady and a dad who came home every night predictably at 4:30 p.m. after work. She could plan on a regular schedule, count on sleeping in her own bed, and know that she would be hugged every night and every morning. She looked forward to our bicycle rides together, learning to drive in an old Volkswagen bug in our yard, going to the nearby lake for a swim, and having food on the table that I cooked, however poorly, with my own hands and heart.

But now, as she rode with Uncle Bill, after a normal day at school, suddenly she wondered what was happening to her. I always came home to cook dinner and put her to bed.

A few days later, after appeals from her Grandmother, Carrie moved to Grandma's house. Grandma's house was closer to the hospital where I was. She thought maybe life would return to normal, and I would get better soon.

Carrie's time with her mother had not taught her anything feminine. And my motherly approach to buying clothes for my daughter was that of a typical male. For example, when I took her to Sears to purchase her first bra, I turned her over to a saleslady in the Girls' Department and asked the saleslady to help Carrie select a bra. Since I had no idea how to determine the correct bra for her.

When she arrived at Aunt Linda's home and congratulated herself on hitting the jackpot, Carrie was jolted by the fact that she faced a life completely different from being raised by me. Her cousins were well-trained by Aunt Linda, and they took seriously the task of teaching Carrie how to clean, how to keep a room neat, how to wash clothes, how to iron, how to do dishes, and how to cook. Carrie began to wonder if she was living the life of Cinderella.

Carrie learned a lot, but she had none of the privacy she had grown accustomed to in her own room on the edge of the forest with Lady and me. She had no one that gave her unwavering devotion like Lady; in fact they had no pets.

As soon as I showed signs of some recovery, and thus it was safe for Linda to go back home for periods of five or six days, it became clear that Carrie and Aunt Linda were like oil and water.

It was a full two months before Carrie visited me in the hospital. I was just regaining the ability to move both eyes, and I was on the verge of moving small muscles in my temples and jaw. I still was hooked to the breathing machine, catheter, and feeding tube, and tubes were in my legs where permanent cut-downs had been done so medical staff could mainline medications into me without having to find my collapsed veins in my arms.

Upon her arrival at my hospital room the first time, Carrie was very nervous. She was excited about finally seeing me. The most overwhelming thing for her, however, was the odor of the hospital. But mostly it was the shock of seeing me helpless and paralyzed that was hard for her.

Carrie visited me several more times while I was at the hospital. But her best and longest visits took place after I had been moved to a hospital near her. By then, Carrie had finished the school year and was more comfortable in her home setting.

Once I had moved to the new hospital, and once Carrie was comfortable with having her own room and a new school, I could see her more often. I even could begin to think about a rehabilitation hospital that would help me return to life outside the hospital by teaching me to feed and dress myself while only having slight use of my hands, arms and legs.

My move to the new hospital, while hooked to a breathing machine in an ambulance, was the real start of my recovery process. Although I had regained some movement at the previous hospital, there was no planned effort to get me the therapy I needed to recover and restart my life outside a hospital.

Chapter V

Night 1 – Welcome to ICU

I would hate to know the statistics about the number of people who die in hospitals around the world each year because patients weren't heard or listened to. The figure must be staggering. I was nearly such a statistic several times. My first two weeks in the hospital were like a trip to a torture chamber, not the professional medical care seen in a TV sitcom. There was no doctor with a magical cure.

Night One was a foreshadowing of what was to come.

A nurse came into my room, and without a word of explanation opened my mouth and began shoving what felt like a big plastic tube down my throat. I was failing so rapidly that I couldn't raise an arm to defend myself. I was dumbfounded. Why was she doing this? Was this something to help me? Was she trained at the Marquis de Sade School of Nursing?

Then I heard a voice, when it was impossible for me to answer because of my paralysis and because of what was being forced down my throat. It was another night shift nurse walking up and telling me that the medical staff was worried about my throat closing and restricting my breathing.

If I had been given a chance to tell them, I would have said, "You are wrong." My strength was failing, but I had no swelling in my throat. No one had checked on my breathing. What doctor would order anything for a patient without some test or physical examination?

I gagged on the tube, too weak to resist, protest, or spit it out. Confused, I spent the night in great distress, wondering what was happening to me as I breathed through the plastic tube.

I wondered was this an isolated incident?

Night Two in ICU answered that question when the night shift personnel had to change my bed. By then I was unable to move anything but my left eye, and I quickly learned that the staff members were not aware of the need to watch my eyes for signals I might try to send. Being helpless, I could only lie and endure the pain they were about to inflict.

The nurses asked my sister to leave the room.

With my sister safely outside so she could not witness what was to happen, and because I could not speak (thus not likely to cry out or report what was about to happen), the two nurses rolled me on my side against the bed rail. Thus they could make the half of the bed that I no longer occupied. Then one nurse draped one of my arms and one leg over the side rail of the bed. She grasped an ankle and a wrist, and with one of her feet braced against the bed, she pulled hard to keep me from falling back on the bed while on the other side the nurse rolled the old sheet as far under me as possible. She then made that half of the bed with a clean sheet, pushing what remained of the new sheet under me with the old sheet.

For a normal person this wouldn't be a problem, but with no control of my muscles, the pain was excruciating. I had no muscle strength to resist her yanking on my arm and leg, thus protect my joints, and the nurses seemed to assume that because I was paralyzed, I also had lost feeling and the ability to sense pain. Or they simply didn't care. My arm and leg were literally being pulled out of their sockets. After one half of the bed was made, releasing the arm and leg, they allowed me to fall onto my back into the middle of the bed, rolling over the half of the sheets tucked under me.

Less than a minute later, they rolled me over to the other side of the bed. Then they pulled me up onto the other side rail to make the second half of the bed. My head flopped, as I had no control, to that side. I was staring at the nurse. She was showing no emotion. She again gripped my other ankle and wrist, again draped over the bed rail, and with one of her feet braced against the bed, the nurse pulled me against the bed rail while the other nurse pulled out the old sheet and threw it on the floor. The new sheet was pulled out and the remainder of the bed was changed. After they finished making the bed, the nurse holding my ankle and wrist simply let go. Dropping me like a sack of potatoes, and I rolled to the center of the bed. The nurses then straightened my head, legs and back, leaving no evidence of what they had done. The linen change finally was accomplished, and they left the room, apparently with no thought of how their job had affected the patient, me.

I couldn't speak or move to let them know how much pain I was in. Not one word was spoken to me by the nurses. In addition to the pain, there was the humiliation of being treated like nothing but an inconvenience that somehow had gotten in the way of the conversation these two had begun at the nursing station a few minutes earlier.

I soon realized that changing the bed would be a nightly ordeal. I needed my family to instruct the staff on how the routine changing of my bed would be done.

The light at the end of a tunnel usually signals a way out of a bad situation or a train coming and there will be more trouble. This experience and other ICU experiences made it seem as if there was always a train at the end, and the tunnel was a hospital hallway leading to my room. In the beginning it appeared as though my situation would never improve and mistreatment never end.

I'd be forever in a hospital bed, paralyzed and at the mercy of a hospital staff that seemed to be somewhere between ignorance, indifference and sadism, depending who was treating me. The terror of being paralyzed and being so poorly treated by some of the hospital staff made me think about the negative possibility of my future, without communication to the world outside of my body.

I was going downhill very fast. After only two days, I couldn't breathe on my own. The tube down my throat was replaced with a tube up my nose to which a respirator was attached.

When I was first connected to the respirator, I was told not to fight it. Imagine air being forced into your lungs. The natural response is to force air back against the incoming pressure to protect your lungs, rather than relax and let a machine breathe for you. The first hour that I was connected to a respirator was a battle. I would try to take a breath; the respirator would try to force air into my lungs. Every time I took a breath, the machine let out a loud screeching noisy alarm.

Eventually I tired and became too weak to fight, and the respirator won the battle and began breathing for me. It would continue to do so for the next eight months, but I never got comfortable with the fact that a machine was breathing for me.

The steady thump, thump, thump sound of the breathing machine became a taunting. It sounded to me as if it were a terminator with a hatred for humans like me that it felt had no use.

In the beginning, the respirator was connected through my nose. The nose is a very sensitive organ. I learned the hard way just how sensitive.

It was bad enough to have a hard plastic tube forced into my nose and down my throat to connect the respirator, but, to make matters worse, the tube took on an evil life of its own with each inhalation and exhalation. Air was forced into my lungs to fill them, and then a valve allowed the air to escape through the same tube. Each action moved the tube in a different direction. This was repeated ten to fifteen times per minute, and it continued without relief. It was as if someone was twisting, then pulling on my nose. Then, as a bonus, a "sigh" was mechanically introduced into the breathing cycle every couple of minutes. A respiratory machine "sigh" is an extra-large volume of air forced into a patient's lungs to fill the lungs completely.

The continuous movement of the plastic tube became a torture that went on for ten days. During the first week my entire nose became raw and sore. All of the rubbing had taken its toll. Each time the respirator pumped a breath, I felt a stabbing pain to my nose from the rubbing back and forth. The sighs were something I especially dreaded because the extra pressure moved the tube more violently. It was as if someone was grabbing my nose, then twisting it. The sighs came at regular intervals, preceded by a noise that sounded as if the machine was preparing to work harder. That noise put me on edge every time I heard it; I knew about the pain that was coming as my nose was about to be distorted and ripped. Sleeping became impossible; if I dozed off, the pain from the respirator would immediately awaken me.

When things got bad enough, I asked to have my throat slit to relieve the pain in my nose. Actually, I was asking the medical staff and my family for a tracheotomy, because I needed relief from the pain.

A tracheotomy tube would be inserted surgically through the base of my neck and into my throat. A balloon around the tube would seal off my throat, so the tube would bypass my nose and mouth on its way to my lungs. In effect, my mouth would be disconnected from my lungs and stomach. I wasn't going to eat or talk for a long time, so I calculated that the loss would easily be offset by the elimination of the constant and intense pain to my nose.

Finally, the day after Christmas, I got a tracheotomy as a belated Christmas present. Coming out of surgery, I was asked by my family what they could do to help. My eye-rolled answer: "Big Mac and shake. "

It was my special brand of humor.

It felt so good to have my nose back—no longer twisted and rubbed raw by the plastic air tube. So, I was letting my family know I was feeling better. Sick humor from a sick man.

Although I was free of the constant pain from the nose tube, the respirator still was my nemesis. That breathing machine came with a Respiratory Therapist, whose job it was to maintain the machine and perform some procedures on patients connected to it. One of them was incompetent. He seemed to be oblivious to his patients as he did his nightly chores.

His task in my room was to clean my respirator, in order to insure the air going into my lungs was not contaminated with mold or germs.

During the cleaning process, he had to turn off my respirator to pull tubes, clean, and replace any dirty filters. Despite the reality that I couldn't breathe on my own, he would say, "Hold your breath." How could I hold my breath when I couldn't breathe at all? He, a trained professional, just didn't understand the situation, or the effect on me.

Hold my breath?

If only I could....

As soon as the respiratory therapist turned off the respirator, the weight of gravity on my chest forced my lungs to collapse, so the air left my lungs. With no air in my lungs, I felt like I was under water, having exhaled and with no way to inhale. My lungs burned for air. My body tried to fight for air, but being paralyzed, it was impossible to get even a small breath or cry out for help.

By the end of his daily chore, with my lungs empty of air for several minutes, I could see the darkness slowly narrowing my field of vision as I was sliding into unconsciousness, only to be revived when the respirator was reconnected and began pumping air back into my lungs.

I didn't understand why didn't he use a simple and humane option that the other respiratory therapist used? All he had to do was ask a nurse to assist him and "bag" me while he cleaned the machine. ("Bagging" is manually forcing air into a patient's lungs with a small football-shaped rubber bladder attached to the tube in the patient's throat. Squeezing the bag manually forces air into the patient's chest and fills the lungs.) I thus could have breathed while my respirator was disconnected so it could be cleaned. Surely he had the same training as the other respiratory therapists.

I never got a chance to ask the respiratory therapist why he thought so little of his patients that he would cause them to suffer a torture that today would be equated with water boarding. I'll talk about that next. He supposedly was a trained medical professional—but he seemed to have understood nothing about his job except its mechanical aspects. A robot could have performed as well. I often have wondered if any of his patients died while he ignored them and the misery he caused. And if they did, how he covered up his incompetence.

In addition to the incompetent respiratory therapist, the respirator itself was a problem. The respirator led to one of the most repeated tortures I had to endure, which was dumping water into my lungs.

A few drops of water inhaled into a person's lungs causes distress, violent coughing. It is called water boarding. If drops of water can do this to a prisoner, imagine what several ounces of water did to me when they were poured directly into my lungs.

I could feel everything, even though I couldn't move. I would lie paralyzed, watching moisture collect in the sagging tube that ran from the respirator three feet to the hole in my neck. After a few times I knew that it was only a matter of time until all of that water would end up in my lungs. How I wished that I could reach out to disconnect one end of the tube and allow the water to empty into a basket. I'd be saved from the coming torture. But of course reality trumped my mental fantasy reaching out and draining the water from the tube. The respiratory therapist was in charge of my respirator and its tubes, not I.

As the respirator forced air into my lungs, moisture automatically was added to the air so my lungs would not dry out. Because the air was heated before being delivered to my lungs and the air outside the tube was cooler, some of the moisture in the air would condense at the low point of the clear plastic tube. Visualize the tube hanging in a gentle loop between my bed rail and the respirator. The gradually increasing weight of the accumulating water in that low point of the tube caused more and more sagging, and whenever someone moved me, the tube would stretch out straight until the sag was gone, gravity would cause the whole puddle of water to flow to its new lowest point.

The result? Water ran into my lungs in a silent and drowning gush. I would lie there watching it happen and not be able to stop it. Almost as in slow motion, I would see the tube stretch and straighten out, the water start as a trickle, then a stream of water, flowing directly into my lungs. The distress of water being poured into my lungs was misery – a kind of horror film – I was drowning in my hospital bed on dry land.

Once I eye-rolled a message to family members about the water being dumped into my lungs, they alerted the respiratory therapist staff. But the rest of the hospital staff would forget sometimes, and if a family member was not right on top of the situation, someone would move me, and I would get the water torture all over and over again.

Changing my bed and medical procedures all were frequent causes for the water to pour into my lungs. For weeks, it was a daily horror that I would endure. I just wanted it to stop.

Then, to add insult to injury, the water dumped into my lungs had to be suctioned back out of my lungs. This meant that another tube had to be pushed into my nose, down my throat and deep into each lung to suck out the water that had just been dumped there. The suction also removed the air with the water. The suctioning process was painful and air was being blocked from getting into my lungs while the vacuum tube was moved up and down, in and out, of each lung, taking out any air along with the water.

I don't know which was worse, the pouring in or the suctioning out. My body wanted to vomit to get rid of the irritation in my lungs, and sneeze to clear my nose. But all of my muscles were paralyzed, and I could do nothing but feel my body try to heave up and down as my face turned deep red.

Family members who were at my bedside tell me they still can remember the terror in my eyes as I watched the water rush from the tube into my lungs. Then the suctioning of the water back out of my lungs.

A similar demon haunts me yet today, thirty-five years later. Because not all of my muscles have returned to full strength, even now, I must be very careful when I drink. From time to time I will aspirate a small amount of liquid or food into my lungs. And the memory of the water torture returns. This time, along with the memory, I also get a self-defense mechanism that shuts down my throat to protect my lungs and I can't breathe. The muscles controlling the closing of the throat returned much stronger than the muscles opening the throat to breathe, so I wheeze, choke and fight for air just as I did over and over again while in the hands of the medical professionals who were ignorant. People around me panic as they think I'm choking and have to be stopped from trying to help and making it even harder for me to catch my breath.

As a side effect of being connected to my respirator, I picked up a "hospital bug" that led to pneumonia in one of my lungs. A doctor, whose specialty is Pulmonary Medicine was called in to evaluate, diagnose, and treat my new problem. It had been only three days since I had the tube moved from my nose to my throat. Although at the time it surprised me, I would later learn pneumonia is a common disease picked up in hospitals. In fact, it is deadly to the elderly, who are bedridden.

The pulmonary physician ordered that two separate antibiotics be pumped into my bloodstream from a needle in the top of my hand. As the antibiotics struggled to gain the high ground, my temperature was spiking at the same time my heart was hitting

117 beats per minute. So, pneumonia was added to my medical problems.

While I was in this precarious condition, the medical staff ordered X-rays.

X-rays became a common thing for me during my first two weeks in ICU. They were ordered to check my lungs for pneumonia and they were ordered every time my feeding tube was changed. Since I couldn't eat, a tube was inserted through my nose into my stomach. It supplied nourishment similar to baby formula that I would live on for the next seven months. Sometimes when the nurse inserted a new feeding tube, the plastic hose accidentally went into my lungs instead of my stomach. The X-ray would catch this. I could feel the tube when it was in my lungs, but the medical staff never thought to ask me where it was. Instead, another X-ray was ordered. I couldn't help but wonder if the routine was a money-maker for the hospital. I had no way of determining if a procedure was necessary.

Whenever it was time for an X-ray, a Radiology Technician rolled a portable X-ray unit into my room. Then he asked a nurse to help. Together, they rolled me onto my side, placed a hard photo plate under me, and then rolled me onto the plate. The plate was sharp-edged and hard, and it bit into my flesh in the middle of my back with its squared edges pressing into me. The only padding that could be used was a pillowcase. Luckily, the plate was under me for only a short period of time.

To me it seemed like any pain that could happen because of the breathing machine, happened to me. Like Pleurisy. Pleurisy is inflammation of the thin layers of tissue covering the lungs and the chest wall. The outer layer lines the inside of the chest wall, and the inner layer covers the lungs. The tiny space between the two layers is called the pleural cavity. This cavity normally contains a small amount of lubricating fluid that allows the two layers to slide over each other when we breathe.

I don't know if it was from some bug in the hospital, or just my inactivity, but of course I got it. Because I was connected to the breathing machine, every breath was painful, and every mechanical sigh exponentially increased my pain as the two tissue layers rubbed together. I would lie there knowing that a sigh was coming, and I would brace for the pain. There was nothing that could be done except wait for the pleurisy to heal. Pain medicine never seemed to be an option available to me. Eventually the pleurisy healed and pain caused by the sigh from the respirator became a memory in a long list of bad memories that I endured in my hospital stay.

Also on the same day as the X-ray the neurologist came into my room. He had done a spinal tap a few days previously. He spoke to my sisters and me, saying that my spinal tap analysis showed excessive protein in my spinal fluid. Therefore, he thought the problem was Guillain-Barre Syndrome, and I was still on my way downhill and there was no medicine or procedure that could prevent the disease from running its course. All I could think is that this Hell was like a runaway train and it was going to get worse. The one good thing he said was that communication and stimulation were vital, and that the presence of family could be very helpful.

At least now my Hell had a name – "Guillain-Barre Syndrome." He reiterated that there was nothing the medical team could do to stop the progression of the disease. Adding nor could he tell me if I'd survive.

My hope of a quick and full recovery and that the medical staff were super heroes capable of vanquishing all diseases, evaporated that day.

As my time in the hospital wore on, the bed gradually became my enemy. It, even more than the ICU, was my prison. I could see "the world outside" only through the bars of the side rail. Because I am so tall, the foot of the bed had been removed. And with the head of the bed elevated, I would slide, inch by inch, out of the bed feet-first without anything to stop me. These ineffectual and almost humorous escape attempts were always caught by my prison guards before I made it to the floor. In my imagination if I hit the floor, I could escape. Like a prisoner fleeing a dungeon, I would be free if I could just make it to the floor.

To get me back where I belonged, the foot of my bed was elevated above the level of the head of the bed. Once my feet were higher than my head, the edges of the sheet near my head were gripped by two nurses and aided by gravity. Down I'd come, dragged back to the head of the bed like a prisoner being put back in his cell. There I lay again, looking at the world through the bars of my side rail.

Fire alarms made my bed even more of a prison. Because I was totally dependent on my respirator, the periodic howl of the fire alarm scared me. As an electrician, I knew a fire could easily kill the electrical power, my respirator, and then me – in precisely that order. I had thoughts of being a marshmallow, roasting as the hospital burned down because I couldn't leave the room. Luckily the piercing howls all were false alarms or testing of the fire alarm system. But late at night, the only time the alarms went off, I was left with unwanted thoughts, is this the real thing? Or just a test/false alarm. ...

My first time out of bed would not come for months, but when it did, it was one of the landmark moral victories as I left the prison of my bed on the road to recovery.

My first week in ICU wasn't all doom and gloom. It did have some humorous moments. Moments that took me away from my misery and brightened my spirit, even if only for a few moments. Like ....

The time I got quite an education in what some women talk about because two of the nurses thought I was not conscious. I was a ghost they couldn't see. Therefore, they said things in front of me that they would never have said if they had realized that I was alert and listening.

It started as a dark and dreary night, and two small-town nurses were changing my bed while I was in it. They took their time to change my bed, so as to have more time to talk to one another.

One nurse told the other about an affair she was having with a married doctor at the hospital. I never knew how graphic girl talk could be. The nurse described in detail how she regularly met the married doctor for an affair. Late at night, she explained, the hospital was mostly deserted. The doctor would leave his home and his wife and would come to the hospital on the pretext of seeing a patient. The nurse would slip away from her duties while another nurse watched her patients and prevented the supervisor from knowing anything was going on.

Doctor and nurse would meet in a private empty patient room in the hospital where they could be alone. She said he liked the way she showed her passion. She would get him excited by kissing him and slowly running her hands over him. The doctor's wife, the nurse explained, was cold and just wanted the sex to be quick and over. The doctor told her how he loved her and the way the nurse would do anything to please him. The doctor said her knowledge of anatomy helped bring him to levels of pleasure he knew only with her. How he looked forward to their meetings and longed for more of them. She described how sometimes they would slip into the shower and she would use the soap to lather him up, rinse him off, then kneel in front of him to perform oral sex. The nurse said it always ended with the doctor professing his love and the nurse changing the bedding. But it wasn't the normal hospital bed change she did for patients; she had a warm glow about her, remembering how the bed got soiled.

I was struck by how inventive she and her doctor were, and how proud she was to tell her fellow nurse about her unique medical expertise.

The nurse said her doctor was going to leave his wife for her because of the great sex. Strangely, it seemed to me that she described the experience as if it were more a conquest than a love affair. When she talked about the doctor, her focus was completely on how she wouldn't have to work anymore. She would be "marrying up" and improving her station in life. There was no mention of love for the doctor or anything admirable about her doctor. This was my second education: I naively thought all nurses joined their profession to help people. Maybe some are just looking for a doctor to marry.

An irony struck me years after I got out of the hospital. The abbreviation for Intensive Care Unit is "ICU." Pronounced "I see you," the abbreviation should note careful observation. But, like the two nurses talking in front of me, few professional medical practitioners actually saw me. I was more a ghost than a flesh and blood human with feelings. It seemed to me, I was merely a patient; therefore, I had no feeling, emotions, or rights. I couldn't move and speak; therefore, I didn't exist.

Chapter VI

Time, Too Much Time

During the previous two weeks in the ICU, I learned many lessons about life and death, and I realized the danger of having too much time to think.

My second week in the hospital included Christmas Day, and as that normally joyous day approached, I thought of my daughter. I regretted how I was failing her.

I wanted Carrie to be happy and have a stable home. I was no longer able to give her those things. I sent a note to be delivered to her:

"Dear Carrie: Merry Christmas. Hope you like the new Atari game.

Love Dad – I love you."

I had bought her an Atari game set before I had gotten sick and hid it away to be given to her for Christmas. Atari was all the rage that year. I had planned to connect it to the television after she went to bed Christmas Eve, then wait to see the joy on her face when she discovered it....

My note, dictated with eye-rolls, lacked the emotion I felt for her and my disappointment not being there for her. I meant what I said, but what was an 11-year-old supposed to do with such a message? She barely could comprehend that I was going to be in the hospital a long, long time, and here I was dictating with eye-roll code a message about Atari, one of the earliest computer games. How was she making sense of the chaos we all were facing? Our world was being torn apart. What was Christmas like for her away from home and me?

Lying paralyzed in a hospital bed gives a person too much time to think. Besides thinking of the needs of my daughter, I began to analyze my life. My life did not flash in front of my eyes. Instead, it was like a movie being played in slow motion.

Some of the time I thought about how I got Guillain-Barre Syndrome. I remembered that just before I became sick I had torn apart a transformer at work in order to get a machine up and running. I didn't have the parts necessary, and the repair had to be completed fast in order to regain some lost production time. As I rushed, I got some PCB on my hands. As an electrician, I knew that transformers use PCBs for insulation. And from the news I knew it could be a health hazard. Could it have been the contact with PCBs that had caused my paralysis?

My doctors couldn't answer the questions. Still trying to figure out what had caused my sudden paralysis, a family member suggested that my paralysis might have been caused by having a dog in our home. My reply to that was to spell out slowly "H-o-r-s-e m-a-n-u-r-e."

After all that thought, and no answer about what caused the disease, the answer fell into my lap a decade later. In 1991 the Veterans Administration published a list of diseases caused by Agent Orange. On the list was Peripheral Neuropathy.

Peripheral Neuropathy is a family of diseases, and Guillain-Barre is a member of that family. Having spent my tour in Viet Nam in the I Corps, where millions of gallons of dioxin were sprayed to kill the jungle foliage, I knew I had been exposed to Agent Orange. I learned later that the Veterans Administration does not dispute that fact. During the siege at Khe Sanh, the only water we had for drinking over a four-month period was from a river at the foot of a hill I was on. Operation Ranch Hand was the spraying of Agent Orange in Viet Nam. Operation Ranch Hand documents show that Agent Orange was heavily sprayed around Khe Sanh and the surrounding area, and because heavy monsoon rains created a runoff into the river that was our only source of drinking water, I realized what had happened. Our drinking water had been contaminated with Agent Orange. Years later I tried to contact Marines who had served in the same area as me. Only approximately sixty answered, and thirty percent of them said they had neurological problems. Even if everyone had answered and no one else had a neurological problem that was a high number to all have neurological illnesses. Seemed like too many to be a coincidence.

However, as with nearly everything the U.S. Government does, there was a catch. To qualify for the VA benefits, symptoms had to appear within one year of leaving Viet Nam and had to have been cured within two years. Since the list was published many years after Viet Nam, no one could qualify. Without the VA benefits, I had to sell my home to pay for returning to school, once I had left the hospital and begun to rebuild my life. This seemed to be the typical government bureaucracy. The soldiers used in the atomic bomb testing came down with cancer; however, the government did not admit that their exposure to radiation caused the cancer until after the last soldier had died.

After a week of being paralyzed, in pain and possibly dying, one might infer that my thoughts would have moved to a loftier and more philosophical plane. What is the meaning of life? Is there a god? How had I lived my life?

Sorry, but I worried about a freezer full of food. I had bought a hindquarter of beef. A neighbor and I had raised a pig, butchered it, and split the meat between us. I had raised a dozen chickens. There was enough meat to feed my family for a year. And it all would go to waste if my home lost electrical power. What was I to do? I couldn't even give the food away from a hospital bed.

Were my bills being paid? How was I to get the Sears order I had placed before I was hospitalized? How was I to mail the mortgage payments so I wouldn't lose my home?

Thoughts about going home were illogical because my home was not wheelchair accessible, and no matter how much I wanted it, I'd never be able to live there again. I'd never be able to grip the Sears tools I owned and use them. My life in my home, and my days working as an electrician, were done. My sisters would have to deal with the problems of my bills and the freezer, because being paralyzed in a hospital bed. I couldn't. I could only communicate what I thought was a priority.

As my immobility began to take its toll, my muscles began to waste away. As they did, they often cramped. If I was in one position too long, it became painful. It was impossible to be comfortable for more than fifteen minutes at a time. But no nurse had that much time to spend with one patient, let alone one like me who needed to be turned and moved constantly. The hospital's only physical therapist, whose job it would have been to exercise me, had suffered a heart attack and she had no replacement. My family exercised my arms and legs because the hospital staff couldn't. My joints would have frozen from months of inactivity. The exercise had the side benefit of stretching my muscles, which felt so good. I often wondered what happened to the other patients in the hospital who needed a physical therapist.

As bad as things were, I kept my one eye open to see anything good. A funny experience took place after the ICU staff had bought me a Valentine. It was a three-foot Kermit the Frog Valentine card signed by everyone who worked on our floor. As an additional display of thoughtfulness and kindness, they taped Kermit over my bed on the ceiling. Since I could not move my head to see Kermit, they placed him where I usually was looking, the ceiling.

A day or two after receiving Kermit the Frog, I was to get a surgical procedure called a "cut down." A cut down is a surgical procedure; a one-inch wide incision exposes a vein, and medical staff then could insert an intravenous line. I needed an IV constantly for medicine and in case of emergency, but my arm veins were not cooperating. After two months of drawing blood and inserting IV's, the veins in my arms were hiding from the needles. The vampires, who arrived at night to draw my blood, were having a difficult time finding a vein in my arms. So a cut down was used to get the IV inserted into one of my leg's veins. I still have one-inch scars on my legs from several cut downs.

One day a doctor came into my room with two nurses to perform the procedure. The first thing the medical team did was to turn on the surgical lights located above my bed. As they were busy performing the cut down, they failed to notice that Kermit was covering one of the lights. Of course, I was the only one looking at the ceiling. I noticed that Kermit's belly was getting a small dark spot. As the spot began to grow, I began eye-rolling as fast as I could, trying to get someone's attention. The bigger the dark spot grew on Kermit, the faster and more frantic I moved the one thing I could control – my eye.

One of the nurses finally noticed and asked me what was wrong. I eye-rolled "UP." Naturally it made no sense to the nurse. So she asked me to repeat my eye rolling. I sent another "UP" message. By then little pieces of ash began to fall from the ceiling. The doctor calmly looked up and said "get that out of here" and returned to his surgical procedure. One of the nurses stepped on the bed, ripped the smoking Kermit off the ceiling, and ran out of my room. Once in the hall, she began stomping Kermit – to the amazement of some visitors who had no clue as to why she was attacking the poor frog.

I kept Kermit for a long time, a reminder of both the persistent helplessness and periodic humor that marked my long, long days in ICU. But eventually I wanted no more reminders of the feeling of helplessness and despair that those early days of hospitalization bought. So, Kermit is no longer with me.

It didn't take long, and it didn't take a genius, to see that death was a very possible outcome of my hospital stay.

I had been around death before. When death is near, there is a quietness to the air, almost as if the air is too heavy to move. Then there is the smell. When I was in Viet Nam, I always knew if death had paid a call. I could smell and feel it before finding the bodies.

There were days in the hospital when I could feel Death hovering. As though it was waiting, hiding in the shadows, looking for a chance to claim me, and the only thing I could do was hope he was not given an opportunity. But as I was to find out, like my muscles, it was out of my control.

One of the effects of my Guillain-Barre was that virtually all my body systems would go out of whack. Even the autonomic systems, the ones I could not control, such as body temperature and heartbeat, became wildly erratic. I experienced very rapid heartbeats at times. The heart monitor would begin counting up. I would watch it, wonder how much higher it would go. There was nothing I could do, but hope the rapid heartbeat wouldn't damage my heart and hope it would slow down to a more reasonable number. Something as simple as my arm resting next to my body was uncomfortable because of the heat they generated. I felt like I was burning up. In the dead of winter in a cool hospital room, I wanted only a folded sheet covering only my crotch, only for modesty. If I could have had a window open with snow blowing in, I would have been more comfortable.

I had read about someone who claims to have had a near-death experience. They were fascinating to read about. Then I had one, because of my heart stopping.

The experience I had was neither good nor bad. It just was.

How near death I actually was, is something I can't say. The nurses came into my room and rolled me up on my side. Suddenly, I could feel the world slipping away, fast. So fast that I couldn't eye-roll a warning. As I faded, I didn't lose consciousness, but I knew that I wasn't in the hospital bed any longer. I had slipped into a place that was unknown to me. I was moving down a small tunnel. The walls of the tunnel were multicolored, and my eyes were open, with the soft walls of the tunnel rubbing against them. I could feel the motion, but I wasn't doing anything to be moving, nor could I control my speed or direction. I was being propelled forward toward the opening at the end of the tunnel with no way to stop or turn away. At the end of the tunnel was a dark opening.

Suddenly, before I reached the tunnel opening, I was back in my hospital bed with a lot of worried faces staring at me. I hadn't made a conscious decision to come back; suddenly I found myself in my hospital bed again. My sister later told me the hospital staff had called a code, signally I was dying, because my heart had stopped.

When I was back in this world, I needed to use the bedpan. The nurse told me to just defecate in the bed. The medical staff knew that I had flat-lined, and no one wanted to risk moving me and causing it to happen again until a doctor arrived. When the doctor got there, he wasted no time installing a pacemaker though my thigh. He floated a wire using a tiny balloon, it floated up the vein in my thigh to my heart. The pacemaker itself sat on a table near my bed. The wire floated to my heart was an electrode to stimulate the heart on command from the pacemaker. The pacemaker would keep my heart working until I had recovered enough to no longer need it. Later I was told that my Vagus Nerve, which controls heart rate, was being attacked by my disease. The pacemaker recorded every time it functioned to maintain the heart beating. There were no more flat-linings, the pacemaker did its job a number of times.

I eye-rolled a message to my sister, Diane, who is an attorney, after the pacemaker was inserted. The thoughts were short and choppy because of the time it took to spell out the words in our eye-rolling code. I had to express myself in as few words as possible, yet get the message across. Even a short note like this one took thirty minutes to spell out as Diane jotted my code through her sobbing:

"Make a Will. Make a Will now! If die, throw a party. No funeral. Cremate. Wish I had expressed love sooner. Make a Will."

I was not depressed, it was just me looking at what had happened and deciding what to do next. A Will is something that must be dealt with when death is near. I felt that the funeral and related things, were my responsibility.

Because I am a realist. It was the right thing to do under the circumstances, and I knew that I needed to take care of Carrie, because of the threat that my former wife might want to step in and take Carrie. I knew Carrie would have a better life with my sister than her mother. I couldn't control my body now, but I could control what happened to what was left of my world after death.

After almost two agonizing hours, with errors galore, Diane wiping her eyes and blowing her nose as she took my "dictation," it was finally done.

I knew that my Will would be carried out. Despite the fact that my Vagus Nerve might stop telling my heart to beat at any moment. I had what I needed most. Confidence my daughter would be cared for.

Was I scared of death?

No, but my first few steps to death's door were not anticipated or wanted. There were things I still hoped to do. I had cheated Death in Viet Nam – or had he just waited to collect? Did I want to live a life confined to a hospital bed? What about the future? Would it hold more bad hospital experiences for me? Now years later that I have some mobility, if I wait until I'm too weak to control my body, another hospital or living in an institution would be a nightmare until death eventually sets me free of this worn out body. That is something that I don't want to face again. So today, I have made another Will, this one a Living Will to insure my treatment in life or death situations.

Post-Polio Syndrome is a risk I now must face, years after I have left the hospital. With it is the gradual weakening of the muscles. The prospect of my muscles deteriorating and my returning helpless to a hospital is a nightmare. Do I want to return to life in a hospital? No, thus the Living Will.

Funny – the purpose of my life is not clearer now that I have survived all these ordeals.

Chapter VII

One Eye Is Better Than None

Not long after having a near death experience, I experienced something that made me wonder if surviving it was such a good thing.

My only connection to the world outside of my body was my left eye. No other part of my body moved. I could not blink, because blinking requires eyelid muscles, and my blinking muscles were not functioning. To talk, I used the left-right and up-down movements in my left eye, the only thing in my entire body that I could control.

My eye control had become so weak that my family members and nurses had to use their fingers to open my eyelid in order to see what I was saying.

The only thing functioning, other than my intellect and my feeling of pain, was my sight. So when a male nurse squirted an anti-bacterial jell into my eye, blinding me and immobilizing my one good eye, I was more than panic-stricken. It was like the lid of a casket had closed. Mentally I was screaming and clawing at the casket's lid. But to the world outside my body, I looked like I was resting comfortably. The jell stopped me from communicating with anyone and from seeing anything. I was completely blind and helpless with no connection to the outside world. My world had shrunken to being only my mind. My brother was on watch that night, and he ignored my pleas not to allow the nurse to repeat the application of the anti-bacterial jell. The nurse knew that if I couldn't communicate, he would have an easy last four hours in his shift. I am certain that he knew what he was doing: He was shutting me up and insuring he wouldn't be bothered by any requests from me.

Because I had complained through other members of my family about the two previous days when the anti-bacterial jell was put into my eyes, the doctor on duty had left orders that I didn't need any more of the jell. But the male nurse convinced my brother that I needed the jell. I objected, but neither the doctor's opinion nor mine made any difference. As the nurse squeezed the tube, it appeared to be happening in slow motion. The tube of jell was hung over my eye like the barrel of a cannon. It looked huge because it was so close to my eye. I couldn't turn my head. I couldn't raise my hand to protect myself. I couldn't even close my eyelid in self-defense.

Then a white column of jell slowly flowed out of the tube and into my eye. I could see around the jell until the nurse closed my eyelid and rubbed it in.

Now, I was trapped as never before in my entire life. Not only could I not see, I couldn't tell anyone what I was feeling. I had to lie there knowing the pain was coming. Having experience being in one position, I knew the pain would come long before the male nurse returned in two hours. I listened hopelessly to the clock in my head. I knew that after ten, maybe fifteen, minutes on my side, with my weight pushing into my shoulder joint and hip joint, I would begin to feel the pain begin. Lying in one spot would start the burning sensation because of the pressure. The burning sensation felt just like a lighted match being held next to my skin, and it would not stop until the pressure was relieved.

Quadriplegics and paraplegics know about pressure sores caused by being in one position too long. Pressures sores break down one's skin and leave seeping holes in the skin. The body's warning is a burning sensation to prevent this from happening. This warning tells the body that the pressure must be relieved or the skin will break down. The body, trying to protect itself, doesn't stop sending the warning. The pain only gets more intense until the body is repositioned and the pressure is relieved.

As I heard the male nurse say the words that he would be back in two hours to turn me, I knew immediately I was in deep trouble. Then I could hear my brother walk over to the corner of my room. I knew from the corner he couldn't see my eye, nor monitor me. The chair cushion squeaked as he sat in the corner. I could hear the rustle of paper as he read the newspaper and turned the pages. Then quiet, did he fall asleep for the next two hours? I was trapped in the hospital bed. I could have been on a desert island, for no one would see or hear me during the next two hours.

After a half hour my skin began to burn. The good news was that the burning pain was more intense than the throbbing pain in my shoulder from the weight of my body pressing into the socket, so I didn't notice my shoulder. After forty-five minutes, the burning sensation increased, and it became like a blowtorch was being held against my skin.

It got worse, but there was no one to ask for help. My only voice, my connection to the world outside my body, my left eye, had been silenced.

After an hour the pain became unbearable. In my head I was screaming to move. I tried to distract myself. It didn't work, and the pain was increasing. I tried to meditate, but I was in too much pain to concentrate. I tried counting seconds, hoping to estimate the time to when I'd get turned. I tried listening for footsteps or music, anything that would help me not to think about the burning.

Nothing worked.

Still no one was paying attention. Help was a few feet away, if only he would put down the newspaper, walk over to the bed and ask me if I was OK.

But he didn't.

With no way to measure time, I could only hope that soon the two hours would be up. It was an eternity to endure the ever-increasing, excruciating pain. The muscles controlling my tear ducts didn't work, so I couldn't even cry.

Somehow I maintained my sanity as the two hours passed. The male nurse came back into the room, he turned me over, and put more jell in my eyes to guarantee my silence until he returned. Again, no argument from my brother. My brother didn't even check on me to ask me how I was doing. But at last I had relief from the burning pain in my side. Rolling me onto my other side made the pain stop. The pain was gone, and so was the nurse, saying he'd be back in two hours. Somehow I drifted off to sleep in these few pain-free moments.

I was awakened after about an hour by my body because the burning had returned. Once again, I had no way to communicate with anyone. I felt alone, isolated. In a hospital full of people, my brother in my room, no one knew what was happening to me. It was like being in the dungeon of a medieval castle, tortured and calling out in pain. No one could hear me.

Again the pain began to increase. This time I knew there was an end in sight, but the excruciating pain soon overcame reason. I would need to endure the pain, because I had no other choice. But that didn't make this version of Hell any easier. Eventually the nurse's shift would end. He had had an easy shift, which I paid for with my pain. The next day, with the jell removed from my eyes, I communicated with other members of my family. The episode would not be repeated, they assured me.

Then they raised holy Hell with the entire hospital staff, all the way to the top. And my brother returned home, never to stand another shift of watching me.

Somehow I had maintained my sanity, but that experience, after the near-death Vagus Nerve experience, made it clear to me that death is not such a bad option when things get bad enough. Everything and everyone has limits of what they can endure.

Years later I learned about hospital air mattresses that automatically and continuously inflate and deflate in three zones to shift the pressure points of a patient's body. Either the hospital didn't know about the technology or it wasn't available to them. Too bad. The bed would have saved me that night when my one functioning eye was blinded by the male nurse, as my brother sat across the room reading a newspaper, totally unaware that I was in so much pain for so long a period of time.

Chapter VIII

They Shoot Horses

Reality versus optimism is always a battle. Growing up we are told we can be an astronaut, Major League ball player, President.... But there are few of those jobs available and most of us will not get them.

For the most part, I hoped that I would make a complete recovery. Even in my dreams I could walk, run, my hands functioned and I was happy and pain free. Then one day a nurse came into my room, when my sister took a break and was out of my room. She and her co-workers had discussed my condition and decided I needed to hear the truth, as they saw it from their medical expertise viewpoint. She said matter-of-factually that I needed to face reality; I would never get better. I should prepare myself for a lifetime of being an invalid. Without saying another word, she then turned and left my room, having delivered her message. I am sure she had the best intentions and had no malice toward me. But with my future progress uncertain, her words hit me hard. Was she right? Was I too optimistic? So I reverted to something I'm good at – Math. The doctor said my myelin sheath regrows at about 1 mm per day (assuming no scar tissue or other complications). I estimated that I would need about four to five feet of myelin sheath regrowth. That is about four years or more, if there were no complications, for the myelin sheath to regrow. The neurologist said I could only expect regrowth for about eighteen months. The math said total recovery was improbable.

With that version of reality, I started to think about my future. Did I want a life that would be a struggle every day just to do the simple things, like get dressed, eat, bathe, grocery shopping, or go to the movies? And then there was the pain.... I knew there were no absolute values and that my calculations were based on average statistics, but still the numbers foretold that there would be no complete recovery.

Armed with this knowledge, I made a decision that the long, painful road ahead wasn't worth it. When my sister came into my room, I asked her to unplug me from the respirator, knowing I would suffocate and die. She refused. I blinked out to her "They shoot horses, don't they?" It was perfectly logical to me. My logic and her morals didn't agree. So, not being in charge of my own destiny and unable to reach over and turn off the machine, I was forced to continue.

This lesson wasn't lost on me. Today I have a living will that states no extreme measures are to be used on me. I have no intention of returning to a hospital bed for the rest of my life.

Chapter IX

A New Hospital – and Hope

I had been in the hospital for almost four months, and I gradually was getting better. It looked as if I might live.

Of course "better" is a relative term. I could not move my arms, legs or even lift my head off the pillow. Simple things such as rolling over or breathing were impossible, and I was still on the ventilator, which meant that I was a serious case in the ICU. But compared to my earlier total paralysis, my successful efforts to blink, smile, and move my head side-to-side were major miracles. I was feeling good about my progress, and my new optimism prompted me to hope that maybe my earlier calculations were flawed; maybe it was possible to make a complete recovery in a short time. A positive attitude was essential to surviving my situation, but it was a double-edged sword. It colored my ability to objectively evaluate my new reality.

One thing became clear: It was time for my family to leave. I was getting better; my life was not dangling every minute on the thinnest of threads. And I could communicate more effectively with the medical staff because I could move my head and smile. Since I could move my head, I could activate a call light by having it pinned next to my cheek. And the need for constant watching was much less. Also, the strain on my sisters' families was beginning to show, and they both were needed back at their jobs. They talked to me and explained that they would visit on weekends, and that they would be in touch with the hospital medical team virtually every day by phone.

I was given a choice: Move to a new hospital close to my sister and daughter, or stay in my current hospital without family support. My growing optimism prompted the following thought: Since I was in my home town, and since I was improving, it would not be long before I'd return to my home and to work – life would go back to the way it had been, wouldn't it? Also a new hospital was an unknown. What was the staff like? Since this was my only experience in a hospital, I thought another hospital would be the same. A choice between the devil you know and the devil you don't know.

So, I chose to stay at the local hospital near my home, and the hospital staff was pleased. After all, I had good insurance that covered catastrophic illness. Therefore, was a paying customer (and paying very well, because the cost of ICU is greater than an ordinary hospital room), and my continued stay at the hospital would continue to be a large positive on a small hospital's income. The hospital administration tried to make sure I stayed put, and it was clear to me that everyone got the word: "Keep Sam happy and here." After all, the hospital is a business and needs to turn a profit; it needed paying customers.

At first the nursing staff and the respiratory therapists were very attentive, and only the competent ones were assigned to me. Dawn was an especially good Respiratory Therapist, and I was glad that she had me as a patient on her watch so often. I had gained confidence and respect for her in the past weeks, and I knew that I'd be ok if professionals like her were regulars in charge of my care.

Dawn not only knew her job. She also understood that a human being was connected to my ventilator. She talked to me, even though I couldn't answer her. She tried to make me comfortable when she treated me. Not only did she empty water from the hose connecting me to the ventilator, without dumping the water into my lungs, but she also always made certain that she had a nurse assist her by manually bagging me while she disconnected me from the ventilator. It was the simple things that she did that I still remember and that endeared her to me. Things such as "Hello Sam" when she walked into my room, and "Goodnight Sam" when she left. She understood why not to say "Have a nice day," because it is impossible to have a nice day in my condition.

Reality set in quickly. The number of competent medical staff was limited, and after a few days, a barely competent respiratory therapist was assigned to me on the dreaded 11PM-7AM night shift.

He came into my room without a word, as I slept. The first thing he did was to move the call light switch out of my reach. Then he proceeded to dump water into my lungs – with zero awareness that he had done it. Had he bothered to read my chart he would have known about the water torture that my family had insisted be written for all to see. Did he even realize that a human being was at the end of the tube?

But that would have entailed doing a little more work. When an employee's thoughts are focused on ending the day and going home, the extra effort to read a chart is just more work... something to skip over. Why not take a shortcut? After all, in his mind he was a trained professional that didn't need any inputs on how to do his job.

He then disconnected me from the ventilator in order to clean it. The effort to walk ten feet to the nurses' station and ask for help never entered his mind. As I lay there, unable to move and the call light switch out of reach, I watched him unhook me from the ventilator to clean it. I felt the air rush out of my lungs, and I was helpless to take a breath to refill my lungs. After a short period of time with the lack of oxygen my vision became a tunnel, with him at the end of the tunnel and the black all around him. Finally, the black slowly collapsed inward toward him, my vision went totally black as I slipped into unconsciousness.

Eventually, when I regained consciousness, I saw that Dawn was in my room, and she was bagging me. She had decided to check up on me. I never heard a verbal exchange between Dawn and the male respiratory therapist. Dawn was too professional to have that discussion in front of a patient, but I am confident that she gave him holy Hell.

The next day Dawn called my sister and said, with utterly no equivocation, "Get Sam out of here before they kill him!"

Diane didn't need her to give a lot of explanation; my family had seen enough when staying with me, read enough of my eye-rolled messages, and understood everything that Dawn was not saying. They started the process of moving me to a new hospital. After that night I had changed my mind about staying in the small hospital and didn't argue. The male respiratory therapist had made the devil of staying greater than the unknown.

Thus I began my move to a new hospital in a university town and closer to my daughter.

It was a three-hour ambulance ride, and since I still was paralyzed and unable to breathe, two nurses accompanied me to monitor my vital signs and keep an eye on the portable respirator to which I was hooked. Upon arrival I was transported to my new room in the ICU. At first, it was like being transferred from one prison to another. After I was put in my new bed, the bed rails were raised and I was again looking at the world through bars into an unknown environment to me.

The two nurses who had traveled with me gave the staff at the new hospital a briefing on my medical condition and some facts about me as a person, and my family support system. When they finished the briefing, they left without coming to my room to say goodbye. Maybe they were told to be professional but curt because their hospital was losing a well-paying customer, who would have contributed to their budget for many more months.

The medical service transition started with my feeding tube, which supplied liquid from a tube up my nose to my stomach through which all of my nutrition was pumped. The nurse noticed there was no record in the documentation from the other hospital of the last time it was replaced. So, she ordered a new one. When it arrived, she began pulling out the old feeding tube. It did not come out easily, which surprised the nurse. When it finally came out, I could see that the end that had been in my stomach was caked with old "food." She called in another nurse to witness the condition of the feeding tube and my nose, which took a beating from the size of the gunk caked to the tube.

She told the other nurse that she had never seen anything like it. The tube must have been left in for months, and I was lucky not to have gotten sick because of its filthy and aged condition. My ICU nurse then ordered a catheter (because I was paralyzed, a tube was run through my penis to my bladder so I could pee without wetting the bed). She then had a male orderly remove the old catheter and insert a new one. The orderly deflated the balloon on the bladder end of the catheter, which prevents urine from leaking around the catheter and wetting the sheets. He then removed the old catheter and lubricated the new one before inserting it. After the tube was in place, the orderly inflated the balloon properly.

As the orderly was changing the catheter, I remembered an incident at the old hospital when one of the orderlies changed my catheter. When that orderly walked into my room, I was a little worried. He had a big grin on his face, and he did not look like a person who has had professional training in his job. He began pulling out the old catheter without fully deflating the balloon. It was painful beyond description, but I couldn't cry out. After he had removed the catheter, he held it up to me with the balloon still partially inflated and a big grin on his face... as if to proudly exclaim, "Look I took it out all by myself!"

After the male orderly finished his proper change of my catheter in my new hospital, the Physical Therapists arrived. One of them, named Jane, would become my friend until almost twenty years later, when cancer took her. Jane talked about what she and the other PT's would be doing to help my recovery. But later as I got to know her, it was her ability to see my human needs, that I loved. She arranged for me to be transported daily to another floor, to the Physical Therapy (PT) Department, so at last I could slip the confines of my prison bed.

One incident that I always will remember took place when Jane personally came to get me for a scheduled PT session. This was a surprise because usually an orderly lifted me out of bed into a wheelchair, stuffing pillows around me to keep me upright (because I still had no control of my trunk, and my legs couldn't support any weight, I would have crumpled to the floor). Once the orderly had propped me up in the wheelchair, a "Candy Striper" hospital volunteer usually transported me from my room to the PT Department for my therapy. The day Jane showed up alone and transferred me from my bed to the wheelchair by herself, she also grabbed a blanket for me. When we got to the elevator, she pushed the "Lobby" button, not the button for the PT floor. I was totally confused, but I trusted her. Before I knew it, she had pushed me outside and parked me in the sun.

This was the first time in months that I had felt the sun on my face and the wind in my hair. Too many of the staff in the former hospital lacked this kind of thoughtfulness, making the environment seem to be emotionally sterile. Jane just smiled and said, "An hour in the sun will do you more good than a PT session, Sam. Enjoy an hour of freedom."

Thanks to Jane, I began to feel more comfortable in my new hospital. I again was a human being.

Chapter X
The Vegetable Patch

The ICU in the new hospital had the nickname "Vegetable Patch" among the nurses who worked in the unit. Most of the patients were not conscious. So, the fact that I was able to communicate, my condition was less life threating and required a little less care than most of the other patients, made me less a vegetable and more a favorite of the nurses.

One of the first tasks for me to accomplish in the new hospital was to sit up in a chair. The orderly would sit me up on the bed, then move my legs so they hung off the edge. He then would flop my arm around his shoulder, putting his leg between mine, his foot against mine, so it wouldn't slip, bend his knees and straighten up. Thus he lifted me off the bed and then pivoted me into a chair stationed next to the bed. All this was accomplished with leverage, so he never had to lift my full weight with his back muscles. Once I was in the chair he would position pillows on either side of my body to wedge me in place to prevent me from falling over, because I had no trunk strength.

Since I still was on the ventilator, breathing was a problem everyone had to deal with. However, I had been prone for months, and my heart wasn't used to pumping blood against gravity. The first few times in the chair, I was light-headed and dizzy. But with each session of sitting up I was able to tolerate longer and longer time in the chair. The only bad thing was my feet. Without functioning calf muscle to circulate the blood from my feet to my trunk, the blood pooled in my feet, and the feet turned black. Although it looked bad, there was no pain in my feet from it. So, it was an acceptable price to pay for the pleasure of escaping the prison of my bed and taking a step in my recovery.

One night lying in bed I realized I could lift my left arm. The hand hung limp at the wrist, because I had no muscle to lift the hand, and I had to lock my elbow to keep the arm in the air. Now I had to figure out how to lower my arm, since those muscles didn't work. So, I simply unlocked my elbow and the arm came crashing down on my head. I spent the next hour enjoying the novelty of being able to lift my arm for the first time in months, despite the beating I was giving myself. I am sure any onlooker would have wondered why I continued to raise my arm, only to have it crash down on my head.

The next body part to return was the shoulder shrug. Although my diaphragm wasn't working, the shoulder shrug elongated my lungs, allowing air to rush in, which allowed me to breathe in for the first time in months. Relaxing my shoulders caused me to slouch, which caused my lungs to compress, forcing air out, which allowed me to exhale. By repeating the shoulder shrug, I could breathe. I practiced the novelty over and over, enjoying the fact that I was filling my lungs without the machine. I imagined I was taunting it, like it did to me, when I was first connected to it. I was winning the battle for control of my body. This was only a small victory, but I hoped for many more.

Gradually the Respiratory Therapists removed me from the ventilator for longer periods of time. Sitting in a chair, they would leave me in my room with a nurse outside my room timing how long I'd be allowed to breathe on my own. I had to build my shoulder muscle strength, and I was making progress. It was slow, no overnight jumps in strength. But at night I was always reconnected to the dreaded ventilator because the doctors were afraid I'd stop doing the shoulder shrug in my sleep, stop breathing and die.

I hated the ventilator. It tied me to my room. It kept me chained to my bed and where there always was the threat of water being dumped into my lungs.

One night as I lay in bed after strengthening my shoulder muscles with exercise, I disconnected the ventilator from the tube in my throat. It was a simple thing to do, even without the ability to grasp the tubing. Since it was attached to the tube in my throat by friction and pressurized by the respirator, a little nudge by my wrist as the machine was exhaling created a back pressure against the tube and it would pop off. But like a tattletale, it began loudly beeping to my nurse to be reconnected. The nurse came in and reconnected it, totally unaware that it had not just popped off, as it sometimes did. I figured out that it was the lack of backpressure that told the machine to set off the alarm and tattle on me when the tube was disconnected. So, timing the breaths from the dreaded machine, I disconnected it from my neck and quickly placed it under my pillow to create a backpressure.

It worked!

The next morning the nurse found me sleeping with the ventilator disconnected from me, humming like it thought it was still breathing for me and under my pillow blowing air into the pillow case. I think the nurse understood and had compassion on me, because she didn't scold me or turn me in to my doctor, who would have felt it was too early to attempt to make it through the night without the aid of the machine.

Being off the ventilator for short periods of time allowed me to be in the wheelchair and mobile. No longer chained to the bed. This was both good and bad....

Sometimes things are not as they appear to be. And so it was with the freedom and mobility of a wheelchair without a ventilator connected to my throat.

One day, five months into my illness, a nurse in ICU, wearing her perfectly white and perfectly pressed uniform, became an unwitting accomplice to an old friend: Death.

She had had a brain tumor surgically removed and was back to work too soon. I was later told one of the side effects of the operation was euphoria and it was accompanied by seriously impaired judgment. I noticed her too-cheerful disposition and I was about to experience the impaired judgment.

I knew that something was wrong a day or two before, when she took me for a spin around the hospital in a wheelchair. On a deserted hallway she began to pick up speed until she was running. Later she would say she was just trying to give me a thrill. As we got to the end of the hallway, she attempted to make the 90-degree corner without slowing down.

I didn't make it. I couldn't raise my arm, since that function hadn't returned yet, I had no way to protect myself. I watched helpless to even brace myself for the crash. I slammed into the wall full speed. As I slumped back into the wheelchair, she adjusted my position and giggled, "Wasn't that fun?"

Now, she was the only nurse on duty in ICU, and it was time for me to sit up. An orderly transferred me to a chair, as always. Then he put pillows around me to hold me in place, as always. Then he positioned a call button on one of the pillows so I could hit it with my head to activate it and call for help. Unfortunately, the orderly did not clip the call button to anything.

Shortly after I was left alone in the room, the button slid off the pillow onto the floor without going off. As I watched it happen, I was unable to prevent it. But I wasn't worried because I thought the nurse would check on me periodically. I was wrong.

After I had been sitting there for five or ten minutes, the constant up and down of shrugging my shoulders to breathe caused my weight to shift in the chair. Almost comically, I began to fall over in slow motion. I could feel myself slipping, but I was powerless to stop myself. I was still in the chair, but my side was pressed against the wooden arm of the chair, and my head was hanging down below my waist. A pillow was wedged between the chair and my side, preventing me from falling to the floor. Now I had to force air into my lungs, since the weight of my body pressing against the chair was forcing air out and making it very difficult to suck air in. It was as if I was sitting on my own chest, while trying to breathe.

I couldn't talk, because of the hole in my throat for the respirator. But I could make a clicking noise with my tongue against my cheek. The nurse in the next room either couldn't hear it or was ignoring it. Either way, I was in a bad situation. As I slumped over, breathing became ever more difficult. The weight I lifted when I shrugged was not only my shoulders, but now I was struggling to lift part of my upper body as well. Also, the added weight of my body on my lungs prevented them from filling as fully as when I was sitting upright. And my weight pressing my side into the arm of the chair made it even more difficult to completely inflate my lungs.

I was tiring fast because I had gained back only a small part of my muscles and stamina. In mere minutes it felt as if I had been fighting for air for hours. I kept making clicking noises, unable to shout for help because of the tracheotomy in my throat, and I was hoping in vain that the nurse would come. It was getting harder to breathe. I knew if I gave up I'd die.

I kept asking myself, "Where in the Hell is the nurse?" She wasn't doing her job and checking on me. After a short period of time with each forced breath I took, I started feel Death's breath on the back of my neck. Death was standing behind me, waiting, waiting for me to get exhausted and stop breathing. I could hear Death calling me, and it sounded like the nurses' giggle... "Wasn't that fun?"

After what seemed like an eternity of being slumped over, it was clear to me that only one thing would save me: Stamina. When I became too exhausted to shrug, I'd slip into unconsciousness, stop shrugging, and I would suffocate. Plain and simple. Not rocket science. Just suffocation.

I was near the end of my reserve strength when she finally appeared.

She said, "Oh my God!" Then she pushed me upright and ran out and called the orderly. Although breathing was easier after getting the weight off my upper torso, I was totally exhausted. The orderly came and transferred me back into bed, and he quickly reconnected me to the respirator. He must have noticed what bad shape I was in. When he asked me what was wrong, he sounded as if he were talking from a tunnel and floating farther away from me.

I had used all my reserve strength, and I couldn't answer. I passed out while the orderly was asking me the question.

Since I was not conscious, I didn't hear the conversation between the nurse and the orderly. I don't know what was said, but I noticed that nurse was never allowed to watch me unsupervised again.

Chapter XI

Goin' Mobile

As I worked with Jane, the physical therapist, she noticed that my shoulder shrugging was getting stronger. Using her experience, she came up with an idea to allow me to begin to move myself from place to place.

Jane took some wheelchair wheels that were being stored in the physical therapy department. The wheels that had rims that looked like a steering wheel from an old pirate ship. Of course, the knobs extended straight outward from the rim, and she knew that I didn't have the manual dexterity to grab each knob to propel the chair. She bent the knobs at a thirty-degree angle so I could get more leverage when pushing the chair forward. She made sure that the knobs had all the rubber ends that normally come with the wheels to protect my hands.

She then placed orders that the wheelchair was to always be in my room. After a few instances of the wheelchair getting borrowed and not returned, Jane made sure the entire staff on our floor understood that I needed that wheelchair. I was a bit embarrassed by all the attention on me, but Jane knew the importance of me being able to propel myself, and the wheelchair never again went out my door unless I was in it.

By positioning my hands so the heels of my hands were against the knobs, I didn't need any wrist strength or hand function to transfer my shoulder strength to each knob. A downward shrug propelled me only a few inches at first. By using only one hand, I could turn right or left. Like the WHO song, finally "I was goin' mobile."

Once I had gained enough strength to push a wheelchair, I used it to exercise. But I didn't have enough upper body power to get myself in and out of a wheelchair, so once I was in the wheelchair I didn't want to be transferred out, because I was at the mercy of the availability of an orderly to transfer me. The orderlies had many duties and were not always available when I wanted or needed to get out of bed and roam the hallways and exercise.

Because I was still so weak, I would tire easily and need to rest. So my desire to have freedom from my room required that I sometimes sleep in my wheelchair, leaning against the bed. If I leaned on my bed just right, I could keep from falling on the floor while asleep. My technique became a daily ritual. Using the controls on the side of the hospital bed, I'd raise the bed so that the top of the mattress was just below the level of my head. Pulling up alongside the bed, I would lock the brakes of my wheelchair, and lay my shoulder against the bed with my head resting on top of the mattress. At first nurses would ask me if I wanted to be transferred back into bed. But after explaining why I was leaning against the bed, they understood and just let me snooze.

After Visiting Hours, I was more interested in exercising than watching TV. I was allowed to roam the halls. Normally I couldn't sleep at night, instead I would wheel up and down the halls in hopes that I would get strong enough to be released. One night I went to the Visitor's Lounge on my floor. It had a TV, coffee, and a radio for visitors. I hadn't been able to turn on a radio and just listen to music in almost a year. So, I decided to turn on the radio and enjoy a quiet moment of music.

Unfortunately, the volume control also was the ON/OFF switch. To turn the radio on I had to rotate a knob without being able to grasp it the way most people do. By putting both hands around the knob and using friction in place of my grip, I was able to twist the knob and turn the radio on. However, I wasn't able to control the force I exerted on the knob. To my surprise, and to the shock of the nurses on my floor, the radio came to life at full volume at midnight in a very quiet hospital. I quickly rotated the dial to OFF as nurses came running down the hall. I nearly had used up my favored-patient status in one split second.

One night as I was roaming the deserted hallways on my exercise rounds I came to the elevator. An orderly was waiting for the elevator with a gurney. The gurney had a padded top with cloth hanging down the sides to conceal a compartment under the padded top. In Viet Nam for funerals, we did something similar, but we draped an American Flag over the gurney. Since I was no stranger to such scenes, I asked the orderly if there was a body in the compartment under the gurney cover.

He was reluctant to answer. I think he thought it would upset me that the hospital had lost a patient. But having been to too many funerals in Viet Nam, the sight of a gurney hiding a body was not upsetting. Besides, I didn't think I was terminally ill, just crippled. When the elevator arrived, the orderly took the body to the morgue, and I continued my exercise routine.

The hardest part of goin' mobile was getting back in bed. The nurses couldn't transfer me; only an orderly could. So I had to time my getting from the bed to the wheelchair and from the wheelchair to the bed carefully. I became familiar with the orderly's duties and break times. I got pretty good at timing my requests, even late at night.

The orderlies also gave me showers. Since I could sit up and not being attached to the respirator, I had progressed from sponge baths to showers. As the orderly rolled me into the shower for the first time, I was worried. I still had a hole in my throat and the water from the shower could easily have gotten into my lungs. Even the mist would cause me a problem. Remembering the water torture from the respirator at the other hospital, I didn't want to repeat the experience. The best they could do was a waterproof bandage that did a fair job of covering the hole. The orderly was very careful to protect my throat when rinsing me down. I survived the first one with no problems. Although they were always very careful, sometimes water did find its way to my lungs.

Chapter XII
Food

My first taste of solid food took place on my birthday eight months after I was hospitalized. Surprisingly, I didn't miss eating. It had been so long since I had solid food, I had no memory of the taste.

My doctor was conservative, as are most doctors; his medical practice had exposed him to the consequences of having food go down the wrong way and getting into my lungs. He realized it had been a long time and that I had to relearn simple things, like swallowing. At first he had me eating colored Jell-O, and then had the nurses check the fluid removed from my lungs to see if I had aspirated any of the Jell-O. By the time my birthday rolled around, however, I was moving my head and upper body. My improvement was a result of two things: Time to allow nerve regeneration and muscle strength from all that exercise from pushing my wheelchair up and down the halls of the hospital with shoulder shrugs.

Because the nurses had been feeding me Jell-O, they were aware of my increasing ability to swallow. For my birthday, the nurses asked if I wanted something to eat from the sandwich shop down the street. They were going there for their lunch and would pick up something for me for my birthday. Of all the possibilities, I decided on a hamburger. The nurses went there and ordered one.

Since my hands didn't work, a nurse had to hold the burger and lift it to my mouth for each bite. It tasted great. I was able to only eat half of it, since my stomach had shrunk without being used for so many months. I rediscovered that I loved the taste. It was great to actually be able to taste anything. I paid the price later, because my stomach wasn't used to food that was not a liquid. The upset stomach was worth it, though. I was eating! One more step toward recovery.

The next day, when the doctor made his rounds, the nurses asked if I could start on solid food. He agreed, and neither the nurses nor I let on that I already had begun my new diet without a feeding tube.

After my months in ICU, I was moved and instead of a private room, I got to share a room with another patient. My first roommate nearly got me into serious trouble. Early one morning two orderlies came into our room, I was sleeping and unaware of why they were there. Without a word of greeting or explanation, they loaded me from my bed onto a gurney. At this point in my recovery, I couldn't speak, so I couldn't question what they were doing.

The two men pushed me out of the room and started down the hall. Suddenly a nurse came running up and stopped them. "Where are you going with my patient?" she demanded.

"Back surgery," they replied knowingly, saying they had a chart to prove it.

The nurse looked at the chart that the orderly had taken from hanging on the gurney I was on and handed it to her with a smug smile. She said "This is for the other patient in the room; didn't you check his wrist band to confirm you had the right patient?"

Sheepishly the orderlies wheeled me back into the room and transferred me back into bed. They then loaded my roommate onto the gurney and took him off to meet his surgeons for back surgery.

The next memorable roommate was about my age. When he was first admitted, he seemed to be in emotional distress, but he didn't say a word. I overheard a doctor and nurse talk, I discovered that the man had had a stroke and could not speak coherently. My new roommate knew what he wanted to say, but he couldn't speak words. What came out of his mouth were meaningless sounds. After a while, the man's sister came into the room and told him that his wife was on the way to visit him. The sister stayed with my stricken roommate for a while, and then she was called to a meeting with the doctor, so she left our room.

Shortly thereafter the sister left the room, his wife showed up, and my roommate tried to tell her that his sister was somewhere in the hospital. All that came out was unintelligible sounds. The more he tried to tell her, the more frustrated he became. He was gesturing and pointing frantically, and his wife was becoming equally frustrated, not understanding what he was trying to say. So, I mentioned to the wife that her husband's sister had just left our room to meet with the doctor. The sister hoped to coordinate with her after she learned what the doctor had found out. My roommate smiled, relieved that the message was getting out. He pointed at me and shook his head yes, as if to say that's what I was trying to say.

The idea of having a stroke, at my age, was unnerving. I can understand the frustration of losing verbal skills and control of parts of my body. But I had always thought strokes were an old-person disease. To lose control from a stroke at a young age, was another example of the fragilities of the human body. So many things can jump up out of nowhere and detour a life into a different path.

The last roommate I remember well and he still gives me a reason to smile years later, was a police officer. He had been called to break up a bar fight. The bar fighters turned their drunken anger on him, and they beat him severely. For his efforts to be a peacemaker, he ended up with his face swollen and black and blue, and he had some broken ribs.

By coincidence, the day the banged-up policeman arrived was the same day my father made one of his rare visits. My father didn't visit me in ICU, now that I was disconnected from all the machines and the threat of me dying was a distant memory, he reluctantly visited me after a little coercion from my sister. Since we had little in common and he knew nothing about my medical condition, he began talking about something in his life. He started talking about being retired that he spent his time hunting and gardening. He talked about his hunting experiences and his pleasure of living far out in the country where there were no neighbors. He went on at some length about his recent success in shooting a deer out of season, and he said his wife cooked the venison and it was delicious. I was unable to stop him from talking. After he had boasted a bit, I quietly told him that my roommate in the bed two feet away was a state trooper, who had gotten badly beaten while trying to break up a bar fight. My father suddenly became very quiet, excused himself, and made a beeline for the door. I don't remember him ever coming back to visit.

Chapter XIII

Moving On

The next four months went by quickly. My days were filled with exercising in physical therapy. Jane and Clare worked to build up my strength with the plan to get me out of the hospital. At night I roamed the quiet hospital halls trying to gain strength. Finally, for Christmas I was allowed to spend a trial night at my sister's house. It was to show the doctors I was ready for the next step in my recovery. The bed at my sister's house was a sofa bed, which is much lower than the hospital bed. I couldn't transfer in and out of the bed. So, my family helped to transfer me into and out of the bed. The sofa bed was in the living room. By shifting my weight every hour, I was able to avoid calling out to be turned. The night passed without a problem.

Carrie was ecstatic to have me in the very next room, she probably had the soundest sleep for the first time in over a year. She was overcoming her natural fear and insecurity for the future and my physical presence gave her hope. Maybe, just maybe, I could come and live with her again soon.

After thirteen months in an acute care hospital and my overnight home stay, it was time for me to move to the next phase of my recovery. I was off the ventilator, out of ICU and had no more need for acute care.

I met with a counselor, administrator and medical professional from a rehab hospital. They asked questions to evaluate me. They wanted to determine if I was physically ready and financially ready for the rehabilitation hospital. They checked with my insurance company and found they would pay. The medical professional went over my medical files and thought I was a good candidate. That left the counselor to convince. The counselor asked me what I thought my next step should be. My first thought was to a say trip to Lourdes, France and the Virgin Mary could heal me. But I could see the earnest look on her face, I felt that she might miss the humor and take me serious. I didn't want to miss the opportunity at rehab, so I gave her the answer she was looking for. They were satisfied, so I was admitted.

So I moved to a rehabilitation hospital for the next phase of my recovery with the goal of becoming able to live independently.

The first step on my road to independence was getting out of bed on my own. The rehab hospital expected patients to get themselves to therapy, so transferring from the bed to a wheelchair was the first step.

To accomplish the task of getting myself out of bed with my limited strength, one of the first things they taught me was to raise my bed higher than the seat of my wheelchair. This required that I find a way to push the bed control buttons on the side rail of the bed. Pushing with my finger just bent my fingers, the buttons wouldn't depress. However, by pushing with the heel of my hands, I got the button depressed and the bed to go up. Then I needed a way to bridge the gap between the wheelchair and the bed. They showed me a sliding board, a very smooth wooden board about three feet long and a foot wide. If I could place part of the board under me and the other end on the seat of the wheelchair I could slide my body using gravity, instead of lifting it into the wheelchair. How to grasp my slide board between my two hands that had no working fingers? The staff left me with the board to figure it out. I tried different things and in the end, I found by putting my wrists on either side of the board and pushing in toward the middle of the board, I could control the movement of the board on the wheelchair. Then by leaning over, I could slide the other end of the board under me. For the next step the hospital staff was there for safety. I was trained to position my body on the edge of the bed with my legs dangling. When I placed part of the board under me with the other end of the board in the center of the seat of the wheelchair, I could let gravity do the work. I slid down the board into the wheelchair seat. I mainly had to balance on the board, while falling into the wheelchair. It may sound easy, but balancing was something I was relearning and to balance while I was sliding downhill uncontrollably was a real challenge because of the lack of trunk muscles. Luckily the arm of the wheelchair was tall enough to stop me once I hit the seat cushion. Otherwise I would have kept sliding out of the chair and onto the floor.

Getting back into bed was just the reverse: Lower the bed below the seat of my wheelchair, put the sliding board under me and firmly on the bed. Once I had mastered getting into and out of the wheelchair, the hospital staff left it to me to be responsible for getting myself to Physical Therapy every day.

With the slide board pretty much mastered, the next thing on my "to do" list at the rehab hospital was figuring out how to feed myself. I met with an Operational Therapist, whose job it is to teach daily living. She showed me a leather pouch that secured around my palm with an elastic band. The leather pouch had a place to hold a spoon or fork. I learned to put the spoon in my mouth, then force the spoon into the pouch that I had attached to my palm. My next job was to hit my mouth with the food. At first it wasn't easy. I couldn't control my wrist and my hand started to shake as I lifted the food off the plate. Causing the food to fall off the spoon.

Slowly, I mastered the process that everyone takes for granted after age two: Putting food in one's mouth every time. I had come a long way from not being able to lift my hand, now I could open my mouth, chew and swallow.

One day while wheeling myself to therapy, I noticed a woman sitting in the doorway of her room looking worried. I asked her if she was ok. She said she was waiting for transportation so she could get to rehab therapy, and she was late. I noticed that her arms were hanging limp at her side, so she couldn't push her wheelchair. Transporters were rare or nonexistent because patients are expected to do as much as possible on their own.

I offered to help. I wrapped a long towel around the arm of her wheelchair, and I grasped the other end with my teeth. Fortunately, I had enough strength to pull her to the elevator, onto the elevator, and up to the therapy room. A therapist greeted both of us and started the woman's treatment. After therapy she thanked me and we had a chance to talk.

She had contracted Guillain-Barre Syndrome, the same as me. In her case, onset of the disease began with gradual weakness in her arms and legs over several months. She started noticing being unable to do little things, like putting on jeans. Her husband and children were worried, but they were unaware of how serious her situation was until she fell and couldn't get up. Because of the fall the family called the paramedics and had her rushed to a hospital. There she was evaluated by a neurologist.

She said her paralysis was quickly diagnosed as Guillain-Barre Syndrome, her doctors prescribed a medical procedure called plasmapheresis. It is a process that results in whole blood being withdrawn in much the same way that blood is donated to the Red Cross. The liquid portion is removed and then infused with red and white blood cells. Also it filters the blood, removing disease-causing antibodies.

Unfortunately, this was considered an experimental process and was not available to me a year and a half earlier. It has since proven a successful method for treating Guillain-Barré Syndrome, but only at the onset. The woman and I never developed much of a friendship because she had a full recovery in three weeks and walked out of the rehab hospital.

I cannot help but wonder how my recovery might have gone if I had had the benefit of plasmapheresis. Maybe I would not be writing this while in a wheelchair and still a quadriplegic thirty-five years after onset of Guillain-Barre Syndrome as I was trying to load wood into the pot-belly stove on that memorable day that my life took its detour.

On my way to therapy one day, I heard screaming coming from one of the rooms. That seemed very strange to me. I asked a nurse about it. She said a man riding a motorcycle had crashed and ended up with a closed head injury. As a result of the crash, he was left with the intelligence of a two or three-year-old. She went on to say that he was in a padded room because he would run uncontrollably into the walls and he was smearing his fecal matter on the walls. He was a challenge for the staff. Once he was considered healthy, the acute care hospital had released him. But the family couldn't care for him in his current state, so they placed him in the rehab facility. After a few days, the screaming stopped. I checked with the nurse, the rehab hospital had to release him, because staff couldn't help him function with his limited intellectual ability and the hospital couldn't justify to the insurance company, his continued stay. So, his family now had to either find another care facility or care for him in their home. I often wonder what happened to him. I had been a motorcycle rider for several years prior to getting sick. I remember the feeling of freedom, zooming down the road, the feel of the wind on my face and nothing around me like when in a car and having the body of the car wrapped around me. But I never imagined the consequences of a tragic accident.

Because the majority of the patients in my rehab hospital were suffering from spinal cord injuries, they were young males, who were paraplegics and quadriplegics. This gave them a unique perspective on the world. They divided the world into "cripples" and "TABs." The cripples were us, wheelchair users.

TABs are currently normal folks – <u>T</u>emporarily <u>A</u>bled <u>B</u>odied.

The reality, whether we like to face it or not, is that disease, old age, or accidents await us all. So, I could see the logic in their thinking. These were young men, who thought they were immortal and indestructible, until the reality of an accident, showed them different.

I was caught off guard when talking to one of the other patients, who was in a wheelchair from a spinal cord injury. He told me he felt sorry for me. He said he knew he was in a wheelchair because he screwed up and was in an accident that he caused for himself. But, he said, I didn't cause my loss of muscle control, so I didn't have his sense of closure that he had caused his own future. Instead a random act outside my ability to control, had changed my life that I was now a dues-paying member of the cripples.

On a night I was roaming the halls of the hospital for my nightly ritual of exercise that had become a habit, an outpatient, who was visiting the hospital's Back Pain Clinic, stopped me. Without any word from me, she explained why I was lucky being a quadriplegic. It was better than being able to walk, but having intense and constant back pain, she explained. I was amazed. Since pain was something I dealt with every day. She had no idea what she was talking about and it made it seem a little out of place. Her unrequested and unwanted opinion made me think it was caused by guilt.

I continued to wheel around for exercise at every opportunity, since gaining strength was still my number one priority. Shortly after learning to get into a wheelchair without the help of the hospital staff and the freedom of having no nurse monitor my movements, I decided to take a stroll in the afternoon after therapy and before meals. I went downstairs from my room through the automatic front doors of the hospital, outside and down the sidewalk to explore my surroundings. The sidewalk led from the front door down to the street. At the street the sidewalk split and one way went around the block and the other way went across a street, which had a lot of traffic. The sidewalk around the block seemed like a safer choice. I noticed a slight uphill incline in the sidewalk after I went around the corner. I wheeled as far as I could up the sidewalk that my strength allowed, then stopped and rested in the sun. It was quiet except for the cars zooming past. There was no one in sight. When I turned around to go back to the hospital, that slight incline looked more like a steep downhill ski run to the curb with a drop-off to the street. The difference was the perspective of the incline. Going up was something I could manage. Going down, I could see that gravity would increase my speed until it reached a point, I could not stop.

I hesitated, but I knew no help would be coming to stop me from crashing full speed into the street. So as I started back, I stopped every foot, preventing me from picking up too much speed and losing control of my wheelchair as I traveled down the sidewalk.

It worked! When I got to the curb I was able to turn the corner and return safely to the hospital in one piece.

I relayed the experience to my physical therapist. She had a unique exercise for me. The hospital had a gazebo on stilts, and it rose to a height of about six feet. To get into the gazebo, I had to make my way up a wooden sidewalk ramp that spiraled around the gazebo. It slowly climbed at an incline that a wheelchair could manage. It was a good exercise to build arm strength and endurance. The exercise consisted of pushing up the gazebo sidewalk that spiraled around it, until having achieved a height of six feet and actually getting inside the gazebo. At first I had to stop and rest frequently on the way up and once I got into the gazebo. Later I could immediately turn around and start down. I learned how to use my wheelchair brakes to control my speed on the way down.

I had run an obstacle course in Marine Corps boot camp, but this training was different. I would encounter ramps in the world outside of the hospital and I needed to be able to go up and down a ramp. I managed to complete the exercise, but not without plenty of sweating and tired arm muscles, plus stopping to rest multiple times on the way up. After doing many trips up and down, plus a month to develop new muscles, the trip from the front of the hospital to the corner and back was a piece of cake – steep incline, curb drop-off, and all. And I traveled it almost every day to get out of the hospital and enjoy a little sunshine.

While in the rehab hospital, I had to relearn how to do the simplest things that everyone takes for granted in their daily lives. In the hospital Occupational Therapy began teaching me how to live independently. I was amazed by how little I could do. I needed to learn how to do almost everything because of my limited strength and flexibility. Simple things like how to wipe my butt. Unable to stand, how to pee sitting down in a wheelchair? How could I unzip my pants when I couldn't grasp the zipper? How to cut my food without being able to grasp a knife? How could I ever put on my own pants when I couldn't stand up? How could I comb my hair? Button my shirt? The list seemed endless.

Daily living was something I'd have to relearn to live outside the hospital. I was driven to be a good student and graduate to living independently. Unlike one of the spinal cord patients, I witnessed, he had a hard time adjusting to how his daily living routine had changed. He had to learn to catheterize himself and perform bowel movements manually. He refused to learn. After a few days he was sent home. About a week later he returned humbled and ready to learn, knowing to live independently he would be doing this for the rest of his life.

I still had a hole in my throat from the tracheostomy, it was covered with bandages and gauze. It had been open for over a year and scar tissue had formed. To close it, surgery was needed. One day I was put on a gurney and wheeled next door to an acute care hospital for surgery, then returned to my room when the surgery was completed. The next day I was expected to return to rehab. As I wheeled down the hall to the elevator, I couldn't raise my head. To close the hole, the surgeon cut away the scar tissue and sewed the remaining skin together. So, whenever I tried to raise my head, it pulled on the skin at the base of my neck. I spent the day wheeling around looking at the floor. Eventually the skin stretched and I could hold my head up. I still have the two-inch scar from the surgery. A constant reminder of being hooked to a machine that breathed for me and tormented me.

With no hole in my throat to let water into my lungs, the rehab hospital allowed me to begin exercising in their pool. The therapists were nervous about how I would react to being in the water without the support given by the wheelchair. Being tall and fairly heavy, I would be a problem, if

I panicked because I thought I was drowning. I had always liked the water and was a good swimmer before I got sick, so I saw no problem with me being in the pool. The first time in the pool was an amazing experience. The buoyancy of the water made simple movements easier and I needed less muscle strength. I could stand by holding onto the edge of the pool, a great feeling. I could lift my arms and legs easily. I spent the hour in the pool, just enjoying the sensation of being able to move for the first time in over a year. Unfortunately, it was near the end of my stay in the rehab hospital and I only had a few exercise sessions in the pool.

All the things that would make up my daily life were challenges, and they had to be relearned using tools to aid me. These were the things that filled my time in the rehab hospital, and it seemed as if I was learning a lot of new things every day that I had always assumed would just be done in the blink of my eye. But then, who would ever have dreamed that I would lose the ability to blink my eyes?

My three months at the rehab hospital went by fast, and once in a while I got back to my sister's home for visits. I didn't take advantage of the hospital's driving program because I felt I would make a complete recovery and wouldn't need a handicap-rigged vehicle. Wrong again, but that's another story.

After the three months in the rehab hospital, I still couldn't return to my home in the country. It was evident that I wouldn't be able to live alone, so I moved in with my sister and her husband – and my daughter, Carrie until I could once again live independently.

Chapter XIV

Life Outside the Hospital

I could breathe on my own, feed myself, dress myself, and speak again, a new phase of my recovery was about to start.

I was to be reunited with my daughter at my sister's home, only twenty-five miles from the hospital where I had finished the acute care phase of my recovery. If I needed medical support, the same medical team would be nearby. As an outpatient I visited the hospital, where Jane and Clare were still working with me to help me get to the goal of independent living.

I couldn't return to work; I no longer had the physical abilities to be an electrician. Since going back to my home was out of the question, as much as I loved my home in the country, it was not accessible for me in a wheelchair. College was the next logical choice to regain my independence and my life.

The only hitch was that I didn't have the strength to get a wheelchair in and out of a car in order to get to classes on campus, and there was no public transportation available out in the country near my sister's home. Thus, exercise jumped to the top priority in order to get my life back. I had to strengthen what few muscles I had that the nerves had regenerated, so I could get a wheel chair into and out of a car and thus get started on regaining my life.

My brother-in-law drilled and screwed a heavy-duty eyebolt into a beam in the cathedral ceiling of the living room with a pulley attached to it. A sling was made from a leg of an old pair of blue jeans. A rope was threaded through the pulley. One end was looped to make a seat with the home-made sling. The other end of the rope was left alone for someone to grip and pull to lift me. The sling went under my butt, and the pulley system, because of the mechanical advantage, enabled family members to lift and lower me from the wheelchair to the floor, where I could lie on my back in order to do floor exercises that strengthened my arm, shoulder, hip, and trunk muscles.

To test the system, David, my young nephew, sat on the sling and pulled on the rope until he was up to the beam in the ceiling with the pulley system. It was a simple task to lift his own weight. Having arrived at the huge beam at the top of the ceiling, Dave looked down from his great height with a Cheshire cat grin on his face. His "thumbs up" sign showed us that the sling worked as designed, and it was clear that he had enjoyed the ride up. He rode his personal elevator back down and proved the system worked.

There were lessons for me still to be learned on how to live in a wheelchair. One day when alone I leaned forward to pick up a pencil I had dropped. As I leaned forward, I shifted my center of gravity beyond the front of the wheelchair. The wheelchair with me in it, tipped forward until the footrests were touching the floor and the large back wheels were off the floor. There I was: Balanced on the footrests and the front wheels with gravity causing me to lean ever more forward. I was making a slow motion fall forward out of the chair. I bumped my head into a cabinet that stopped my forward fall.

Unfortunately, the front wheels of a chair are designed to turn freely to make turning corners simple and a shorter turning radius. The split second I was balanced there with my butt in the chair and my head resting against the cabinet, I knew that my fate was sealed; there was nothing to stop me from falling to the floor. The front wheels turned as they were designed to do. My center of gravity continued to move forward as the front wheels turned. My head moved away from the cabinet, now nothing was holding me from sliding forward. Gradually, I slid from the front edge of the wheelchair seat. Until suddenly the wheelchair was propelled backward away from me and the floor came rushing up at me. As I lay there more embarrassed than hurt, I knew I was stuck until someone came home. I lacked the strength to lift myself back into the wheelchair.

Eventually my sister, Linda, who was visiting, discovered me on the floor. Our jerry-rigged pulley system to the rescue. I was hoisted back into my wheelchair as my sister, because of the pulley system, was able to lift me by herself. That was one lesson I didn't want to repeat from then on I closely monitored how I would reach for objects on the floor.

My floor exercise routines were a multi-step process. First a large and smooth exercise board was placed on the living room carpet directly beneath the eyebolt and pulley system. Second, I, in my chair, wheeled onto the board, and the canvas sling was positioned under me as I helped by leaning from one side to the other. Third, I was hoisted upwards a few inches so my wheelchair could be pulled out of the way. Fourth, I was lowered all the way down to the floor. In the beginning talcum powder was spread on the board so I could slide my arms and legs with minimal friction as I lay on my back and side to complete my exercises that Clare and Jane had given me. Since I lacked the strength to lift my body against the pull of gravity, I exercised my muscles by sliding my arms or legs along the board. Gradually the powder wasn't needed and I added weights to my arms and legs as I gained strength. After an hour or so of continual exercise, the entire pulley and chair process was repeated – in reverse.

I did the exercises daily. Never missing a day or quitting early. Finally, I could exercise without being on the floor on the board. I would sit in bed or in the wheelchair with weight cuffs on my wrists. The pulley system was no longer needed and became a conversation piece.

After months of doing exercises I gained enough strength to do something special. This was done only in the summer. I would crawl on my hands and knees down to the lake in back of the house. At first I would only be able to crawl a short distance before lying in the grass to rest. Eventually I could make it all the way without resting. Once I was in the lake I would move my legs and arms freely. The buoyancy of the water allowed me to move more normally than I could on land against gravity. It was like being in the pool at the rehab hospital, except in the lake I was visited by small fish, who came up to me and nibbled at the dead skin on my toes. Unfortunately, I was restricted to days of warm weather. Rain did not stop me, but lightning was something I did not want to be the target of.

Thus were my days filled with ups and downs as I worked to gain strength and dexterity at our home. Sometimes I noticed an improvement in motion or strength and would be happy. Sometimes all the work seemed to provide no results and I would wonder why I worked so hard day after day. But in the end I kept exercising and hiding my depression from the people around me.

With muscles coming back, progress clearly being made, I needed a car if I were to go to college. But I couldn't move my legs, so I wouldn't be able to work the gas and brake pedals. Also, my hands didn't work, so I couldn't grasp the steering wheel. Talking to Jane, my therapist, she suggested ways to drive a car with limited mobility. So, with a little help it was off to the car dealers. As I dealt with them, I realized that selling me a car, any car, was more important to them than selling me transportation I could use. Often the car salesmen showed me cars that they couldn't sell. They thought me an easy mark, since they thought my physical disability also meant I had a mental disability.

For example, I was shown a diesel vehicle that was a putrid shade of orange. It was a four-door model, thus making it unusable to me, no matter how good a deal. (Four-door cars have narrow doors, and being in a wheelchair I needed a wide door to be able to get close enough to the front seat to transfer from the wheelchair into the car.) Still the salesman tried to sell it to me, although I had specifically told him that the car had to be a two-door model. I told him no thanks and moved on to a different salesman.

Another time we had agreed on a car and a price, but when I arrived to sign the papers I noticed that the monthly payments were too high for the price we agreed upon. When I asked to see the paperwork with the price, the dealer tried to make it look as if I were being unreasonable. I killed the deal on the spot. The salesman seemed perplexed that I could calculate in my head that the selling price and the monthly payment were not what we had agreed upon. I don't know what school he had gone to, but I had attended a Catholic school that had prepared me for math and doing calculation estimates in my head.

So, in order to find a vehicle that fit my needs, I again turned to my trusted friend and Physical Therapist, Jane, for advice. She gave me some options that would work. She knew about handicap-converted vans and cars with a rooftop carrier that could carry a wheelchair, and she arranged to have both of them brought to the hospital while I was doing physical therapy. I looked them over carefully.

The van conversion and rooftop carrier were out of my price range, so I ended up buying a brand-new Ford Tempo. A two-door, because the driver's door opened wider than a four-door. (Thus I could get the wheelchair closer to the driver's seat, so a sliding board would reach between them.) The Tempo offered some other benefits, too, in light of my circumstances: I could move the driver's seat forward and back to get my wheelchair behind the seat, and the Tempo offered good gas mileage, which I needed because my only income was Social Security monthly checks. The Ford Tempo clincher was its power steering and brakes and its relatively good price at a friendly dealership, not far from my sister's home. Just what I was looking for, plus an honest car salesman.

As Jane had told me I needed to add hand controls to the car to work the brakes and gas.

My brother-in-law called a boyhood pal and asked him to check the name and address of the manufacturer of hand controls he used. He went out to his car on his crutches, crawled under his dashboard with a flashlight and a pen and paper, and wrote down the name of the hand-control company that had manufactured his car's equipment.

The hand controls were ordered and I was on our way to wrapping up a car deal that would make college possible. In no time at all, I was able to order the Ford Tempo needed, and within a few weeks of my purchase of my new car, my brother-in-law drove my Tempo and my large box of new hand-control equipment to an automotive handicap conversion shop. The mechanics put hand controls on the brake and gas pedals overnight. I was about to take another step forward in my recovery.

But this time I would it would be a huge step. My own car with hand controls to gain the mobility to go to college.

My special gas and brake controls were a system of rods and springs that attached to a lever bolted to the bottom of the steering wheel column, then to the gas and brake pedal. When I pushed down towards the ground on the lever with the heel of my hand, it pushed down on the gas pedal. When I pushed the lever forward toward the front bumper, it pushed down on the brake pedal. When I released the lever, the springs caused the lever to return to its original neutral position and with it the gas and brake pedals. So I was able to control the gas and brake pedals of the car.

Also, the mechanics added a spinner knob to the steering wheel. My hand fit into a metal U-shaped clasp mounted upon the spinner knob, and I could steer without grasping the wheel. All I needed was my hand inside the clasp and my arm strength that I leveraged from my elbow and shoulder.

Next, with Jane's help, we devised a way to get my wheelchair into and out of the car without help from another person. Lacking a butler, I would have to go to school by myself, so I mastered the technique of opening the driver's door and moving my wheelchair as close to the driver's seat as it would go. I would remove the leg rests from the wheelchair and throw them on the passenger's seat. Which allowed me to move even closer to the driver's seat. I could lean into the car and pull the lever at the base of the seat, then slide the driver's seat as far back as it would go to give me more room. I then learned how to place my slide board under me in the wheelchair with the other end on the driver's seat. I thus could slide into the driver's seat. Another good choice for the Tempo was that the driver's seat was the same height as my wheelchair seat.

Now I was seated in the driver's seat with my legs still outside the car, I learned to turn my body so I was facing the wheelchair. I would unlock the brakes on the wheelchair. Then I'd collapse the wheelchair by lifting the seat of the wheelchair by sliding my arm under the cloth seat and lifting my arm up. The wheelchair thus was folded with the front of the wheelchair facing the car. I would then turn the wheelchair around so the big wheels in the back were touching the car. Next I would slide the driver's seat of the car to the most forward position, giving maximum room for the wheelchair to fit through the door, while pinning me between the steering wheel and the driver's seat to prevent the wheelchair's weight from pulling me out of the driver's seat when I lifted the wheelchair. I then tipped the wheelchair so the back of the chair was resting between the back seat and driver's seat of the car. Luckily wheelchairs have handles on the back. They held the chair in place.

Having gotten things lined up, I then would lean outside the car, grasping the wheelchair's seat with my teeth and lift the wheelchair by sitting up straight, utilizing my back and hip muscles – once again using the mechanical advantage and my teeth. This maneuver rolled, not lifted, the wheelchair into the car. Then, moving the seat back as far as it could go, I reclined the back of the seat until it was touching the wheelchair. Next, I put my arms under my legs and fell backwards into the seat, pulling my legs into the car all in one tumble and roll. I then could return the driver's seat to its proper position and my wheelchair was secure in the seat behind me.

To get the wheelchair out of the car, I reversed the process.

Jane was a great help with ideas about how to accomplish my task of putting the wheelchair in the back seat, while simultaneously keeping me from falling as I learned the limits of my muscles' ability. She worked with me as I practiced getting the wheelchair in and out of the car.

I bought the car on a long-term contract, knowing that I needed to come up with money to pay for the loan in the years to come.

Another not-so-small detail....

In order to drive the car, I needed to renew my driver's license. Because I had become handicapped, my old driver's license no longer was acceptable to the DMV. As mentioned earlier, I had not taken driver's training at the rehab hospital, so I would have to learn to drive with hand controls before taking the driver's test at the DMV. My nephew, David, drove my new Tempo and me, with its fancy hand controls, to a deserted road in the country. Driving there he used the hand controls instead of the gas and brake pedals, smiling with pride all the way. After a day of driving and parking, I made the transition from knowing how to drive using my feet to driving using my shoulders and arms.

I was in a hurry to get the freedom of getting into a car and drive somewhere, anywhere. So, without a moment's delay, I called and made an appointment at the DMV, took my written test, then climbed into my car and took the driving test. I passed them all.

Now I needed to sell my dream house to finance my car and college costs. To sell my house, I needed to know its value, so I hired an appraiser. I drove the two-hour trip to meet him at the house. Since I wasn't able to get into the house because of the steps, the appraiser went into the house alone.

As he entered the door of my home, another car pulled into the yard. A man got out, and without so much as a hello he asked if I owned the house. When I said yes, he offered me one thousand dollars cash for the building and land. Knowing that the fifteen acres alone were worth more than that, it took me a split second to realize he was trying to take advantage of me, since he probably equated my wheelchair to a mental disability and an easy mark to cheat out of thousands of dollars. After my experience with the car dealers, I wondered if this was to be a common occurrence, people trying to take advantage of me because of the wheelchair.

When I said no, he went into the house with the appraiser without an invitation from me, and no way for me to stop him. While inside, he asked the appraiser for a copy of the appraisal. The appraiser told me of the man's request. I told him to give me the only copy. On his way out the man gave me a piece of paper with his name and phone number, and he told me to call him about selling the house to him. I destroyed the piece of paper. I hope someday he will be in the position I was and he will understand what he tried to do.

I put the house up for sale. One of the first offers was from a single mother. However, she couldn't qualify for a mortgage from the bank. Fortunately, my sister was a lawyer, and she drew up a land contract. I became the bank for a woman who was down on her luck. The mother and her two small children suddenly had a chance at their own home in my dream house. I understood when they were late or missed payments, something a bank would never have done.

Years later, I'd drive by the house, and I could see that it was in good shape. The two children were playing under the apple trees that had fed Carrie, me, and a herd of deer. I wondered if on autumn mornings they, like Carrie, Lady, and me, ever sat and watched the deer eating our fallen apples. Eventually the mother got on a sound financial footing and negotiated a mortgage through a real bank, and got a little extra money to finance improvements that she wanted. I think my dream home became her dream home.

The appraisal of the house wasn't the only negative experience that occurred because some folks took me for an invisible man in a wheelchair. Much later, when I could drive, Carrie, who by then was twelve, and I went grocery shopping. As we checked out, I noticed that the clerk was only talking to my daughter. When the clerk finished, she turned to Carrie and asked for the money for the groceries. The woman had a jolt and a strange look on her face when I answered her and paid the bill. The thing in the wheelchair could talk!

Another example of how a wheelchair-bound person can be not seen occurred when I went into a restaurant alone. The woman doing the seating assumed I was with someone else, apparently because she believed that a person in a wheelchair could not get into a restaurant by himself. So, she asked other people, who came in after I did, how many in the party? Only when I cleared my throat and spoke up to tell her that I was next did she acknowledge my presence. She apologized and asked me how many in my party and then seated me.

I don't think that most such behavior is done consciously; people just don't interact daily with cripples. Plus, someone in a wheelchair alerts a normal person to the fragility of the human body and serves as an unwelcome reminder that we all are mortal and could easily end up in a wheelchair or worse.

Chapter XV
College Here I Come

I was told that my myelin sheath would only grow back for eighteen months. So, my window of opportunity to return to a normal life was closing fast. I had already spent fifteen months in hospitals, and I was both ready and eager to put my life back together, even if I might not have the full recovery that I had been promising myself.

Now I had transportation, was settled in a home setting with my daughter, and I could think about school. I knew that I would never be able to work as an electrician again, but my mind still worked, so I decided that it was time for me to become employable. Thinking through my options, becoming an engineer seemed the best fit. They were in demand, needed mathematical abilities, logic and their work could be done from a wheelchair.

That meant getting a college degree. I would be thirty-nine years old and competing with eighteen-year-olds. And I would have another disadvantage: I'd be in a wheelchair. My start was at a community college, taking advanced mathematics and science courses to lay a foundation for the engineering degree. Also the cost was much less than a four-year university, which was a major consideration because of my income.

I had not been in a college classroom since 1968. I was more than a little apprehensive about returning to a college campus because I had not been welcomed when I had enrolled in college after my service in the Marine Corps. Viet Nam vets were characterized by the media of that era as drug-addicted baby killers, even though an MIT study would later prove all the media characterizations wrong. In 1968 my English professor assigned our class to write a paper based on a recent personal experience. Naively, I wrote a paper about a Viet Nam experience. The professor gave the paper an "F" because he said the paper had to be fiction and he had requested non-fiction. I explained that it was non-fiction, but the "F" stood. After this experience, along with several similar ones that were due to the anti-Viet Nam War culture that took over college campuses, I was an outcast and not welcome on their campus. I dropped out of college.

Now, as I was recovering from total paralysis caused by Guillain-Barre Syndrome and Agent Orange that I had ingested in the jungles of Viet Nam, I was worried about facing a few more biased and ignorant English professors.

The following quote I hope helps set the record straight about the falsehood of the anti-war bias that pervaded the media and the campuses of America when I was trying to get an education.

From the Nixon Presidential Papers:

Isolated atrocities committed by American soldiers produced torrents of outrage from anti-war critics and the news media while Communist atrocities were so common that they received hardly any media mention at all. The United States sought to minimize and prevent attacks on civilians while North Vietnam made attacks on civilians a centerpiece of its strategy. Americans who deliberately killed civilians received prison sentences while Communists who did so received commendations. From 1957 to 1973, the National Liberation Front assassinated 36,725 Vietnamese and abducted another 58,499. The death squads focused on leaders at the village level and on anyone who improved the lives of the peasants, such as medical personnel, social workers, and school teachers.

Fortunately, in my new college experience I would be graded based only upon the quality of my work. How things had changed. Real education, unbiased education, was the new norm when I returned to college. For example, in a Social Science class, the reading material was about a foreign nation where neighbors were ignoring the mistreatment of neighboring families. A student in my class said that this was just like in America. I disagreed with the student during the class discussion, and I said that Americans were more likely to report abuse than in other lands I had visited. The professor agreed with me.

In the '60s my comments would have been declared dead wrong by many professors because of the prevailing anti-American bias.

To take notes in class I had to grasp a pen with both hands and print, so note taking was slow and difficult. I resorted to audio taping lectures and transcribing the notes later. This made for many late nights, but it also caused me to review the day's lecture and gave me an advantage over the other students, who didn't review their notes.

Winters were difficult in a manual wheelchair. Snow and ice made it almost impossible to move outside. Handicap parking was situated near my classroom building to limit the distance I had to travel in snow and ice, but there were not many handicap parking spaces. By getting to school very early, I could be guaranteed a parking spot. This had the advantage of extra study time, and in the end the loss of sleep by getting up early was worth the parking space. One day I noticed that a man was parking in one of the handicap spots. I was surprised to see him get out of his car and be able to walk normally, almost a run to get out of the cold. I asked him why he had a handicap parking permit. He said he had had a knee replacement and the doctor gave it to him so he would not have to walk too far, since he was overweight and all the extra weight could damage his new knee. The irony is that by parking close to the building, he didn't get the exercise that might have helped him control his weight.

My time at the community college went by quickly. Being older and willing to put in long hours to prepare for class and tests, I usually scored at or nearly at the top of my classes. While taking classes I continued to go to physical therapy, and before I was aware of it, I was graduating with my associate's degree and ready to transfer to a university where I could further pursue my goal of independent living by way of an engineering degree.

Chapter XVI
Learning to Walk

I wanted to walk. I needed to walk. But I knew my desire alone would not make it happen. Because foot drop, balance, and very little muscle strength made it impossible to walk without some kind of medical equipment.

Clare and Jane, two physical therapists, who worked with me, understood my desire to walk and what it meant to me. So they used their knowledge and experience to make it happen. They started with an KAFO - Knee-Ankle-Foot Orthosis. They sent me to the orthotics department at their hospital. There a mold was made of my leg from just above the knee to below the foot. From the mold a custom plastic KAFO was custom made for me.

The knee needs to not bend, because of my lack of muscle strength, I could not support the weight of my body, so I would collapse and fall if the knee bent while it was supporting my weight. Plus, the knee cannot hyper-extend backwards, when my weight is on the leg. So I had to be able to lock my knee to keep it from bending when I put weight on my leg. I had just enough strength to lock my knee, while the KAFO kept it from hyper-extending backwards and damaging my knee joint. Then I needed to have some way to allow my knee to bend forward in order to sit, when I was done walking. Since the KAFO was molded to fit my legs. It allowed me to lock my knee with the top of the KAFO against my thigh and the bar behind my leg below my knee, yet my knee would bend as normal if I unlocked my knee joint.

Similarly, my ankle needed to be immobile in the walking process. Otherwise, my leg would collapse to one side, as my ankle had no muscles to keep it from rolling and spraining the ankle. My medical KAFOs fit under each foot and up on either side of my ankles, up to just below my knees. The sides of the KAFO fit tight on either side of the ankle and preventing my ankles from moving sidewise.

Each of my feet needed to be level when I attempted to raise them to walk. "Foot Drop" is when there are no foot/ankle muscles to keep gravity from pulling the toes and front of the foot towards the ground, when lifted. That could lead to stumbles over carpets and thresholds and uneven pavement outdoors. My KAFOs provided rigid plastic support to the bottom of each foot that prevented my foot from dropping toe first whenever I took a step and lifted a foot into the air.

All this was accomplished using a light weight, but strong plastic. So what little muscle I had would be used to walk, not lift the KAFO.

Jane and Clare next knew I needed some kind of crutches to help support my weight and maintain my balance while standing. They decided on Lofstrand crutches with a special base.

Lofstrand crutches were the solution to my balance problem and supporting the trunk of my body when I stood semi-erect. It was necessary to walk leaning forward to maintain a safe center of gravity over the crutches and KAFOs. Lofstrand crutches are made of aluminum to keep them from being heavy. The base was four legs with rubber tips. The rubber tips prevented the base from sliding when placed on the ground. The base pivoted, so the bottom of the crutch always was stable, no matter how uneven the terrain was.

Since my fingers didn't work, and I couldn't grip the crutches, I had to cup my hands under the handgrips and lift the crutches mostly with my shoulders. The upper arm clasp at the top of the crutches held them in place, not allowing them to slip out of my cupped hands. The four feet at the bottoms of my crutches kept them stable on uneven terrain. When both crutches were on the ground, I supported my weight by locking my elbows and resting the heels of my hands on the handgrips, because my wrists couldn't support any weight. Otherwise my wrists would have collapsed under my weight, causing me to fall sideways to the ground. My weight on the grips, combined with my locked elbows and stabilizing upper arm clasps, formed a three-point stance that steadied my erect upper body, even though my strength in my legs, knees, and ankles were too weak even with the help of my KAFOs for me to stand. In fact, after walking even a little, my ankles would swell up from the stress of the weight of my body and no muscles to support my ankles.

I needed to practice walking over and over to build strength and coordination. Each time I tried to walk a little further. A child falls often when learning to walk, but falling would be devastating to my new progress and new optimism. I didn't have the bones of a child, plus being taller than a child, I would fall a longer distance and with a much harder impact when I hit the floor. A broken bone would mean a six-week delay for the bone to heal. I didn't have the patience to delay my walking lessons six weeks, so it would be a big setback.

So my Physical Therapist, Clare, started the long process of teaching me to walk again. We started in the parallel bars. I would put on my KAFOs and maneuver my wheelchair to the parallel bars.

Clare would put a belt around my waist and use the belt to help me come to standing. I did this by turning sideways in the wheelchair, locking my knees and with the heels of my hands on the tires of the wheelchair, do a pushup. So, now I was facing the wheelchair. While supporting my weight with one arm by locking my elbow, I would swing the other hand over to the parallel bars. With one hand on the wheelchair and the other on the parallel bars I shifted my weight to the hand on the parallel bars. Inching the hand on the parallel bars back away from the wheelchair, I would be standing semi-erect with my weight totally on both hands on the bars. At first I was very unsteady with Clare behind me, steadying my swaying with the belt around my waist. Once I was stable and comfortable that I wouldn't fall, Clare would remove the wheelchair from the parallel bars.

To walk, I would lock my knees back against the KAFO. Then stiff-legged and balancing on the parallel bars and one leg, I would kick my other leg out to the side and swing my hips, so the leg swung out to the side, around and would land in front of me. Then the other leg the same way, all the while Clare was holding onto the belt from behind to prevent me from falling. My gait must have looked like Frankenstein's monster.

I was just learning to balance and coordinate the movements, so I could move a few feet down the parallel bars, a major task. This lasted several months.

More than once Clare would catch me before I fell. But sometimes, when both knees bent, the only option was for Clare to slowly lower me to the floor, because I was too heavy for her to lift me. When we landed on the floor, we would laugh about it and then start over. Clare would get my wheelchair. I would get on my hands and knees crawl to my wheelchair, and with my head in the seat of my wheelchair, put my hands on the seat of the wheelchair and stiff legged do a push up. Then put one hand on the armrest of the wheelchair and shift my weight to that arm, then place the hand on the other armrest. Now I supporting my weight on the armrest, however this was precarious because of the center of gravity of the wheelchair was close to pushing the wheelchair over backwards. Carefully with my elbows locked, then I would twist my body, so my butt was over the wheelchair seat and all in the same motion unlock one elbow and let gravity pull my butt into the seat.

Now back in my wheelchair, I needed several minutes to rest and allow my muscles to regain their strength. Then I once again maneuvered my wheelchair back to the parallel bars to begin the process one more time. Come to standing, inch down the parallel bars, throw one leg out, swing my hips, make a semicircle, and see where my foot landed... I was very careful after getting back up to avoid the mistake of allowing both knees to bend at the same time.

Finally, after several months on the parallel bars, I had the balance and strength to start using my crutches. Then I started walking short distances down the hallway of the hospital on a smooth, flat floor with Clare behind me for balance and support. After several months of slowly increasing the distance I walked up and down the hallways of the PT department, I decided that while at home I would walk out in the street, even though it was on uneven surfaces and without Clare's help. The first time was an adventure, down the driveway to the street. Once in the street I turned right and walked ten yards. Not wanting to get too tired and stranded, I slowly turned around and headed back. In the house and seated on the bed I rested with a smile on my face. The first time in two years I walked outside and I knew it wouldn't be my last.

I was always very, very careful not to fall. All this time I was gaining strength and confidence in walking.

However, despite all my caution in the years to come, I did fall several times. Breaking my leg twice, once so badly I needed surgery and a plate with screws into my leg bone to insure the break would heal properly. I also badly dislocated my elbow, needing to be sedated to reset the elbow. Today, I no longer walk, because of the danger of more broken bones.

Chapter XVII

Onward and Upward

Luckily I now lived near a Big Ten University. I could commute to school and stay with my daughter.

I was thinking that if I could graduate with high grades from a major university, my chances of landing a good job would be greatly increased. My money was limited; I had sold my home, and I was receiving only a small social security check for disability every month with most of it going to pay for school, car payments and maintaining the car. On rare occasions I could afford to take Carrie to a play at the university (being student I got a discount on the tickets).

So I had to get this right, because of my age and financial condition, there would be no second chance to start over. I chose Electrical Engineering. Something I could do from a wheelchair and my experience as an electrician would help and graduates were in demand in the job market. I had finished at the community college. I applied and was accepted into the engineering school at a Big Ten University.

I was surprised how inaccessible the university was for handicapped people. The engineering building only had a freight elevator, but many of the classes were on the second floor. I had to get a janitor to work the freight elevator to get to my second floor classes, because the doors of the elevator closed manually. The doors had a rope to pull the top one down and made the bottom door come up. It was too heavy for me to do and grasping the rope was impossible for me. Some classes were held in the basement of another building, but there was no elevator to get to the basement. I had to reschedule one class for another semester, when the class was in a different place. The only parking for the engineering building was in back of the building, but there was no way to enter the building from the back and no sidewalk from the rear parking lot to the front door. So to get to the front door I had to walk in the street, which was difficult in the winter. And to make the situation even tougher for a person in a wheelchair, parking was extremely limited and there were very few handicap parking spots.

Handicap parking was made even less available by university athletes with leg injuries who were given handicap parking permits. It amazed me to see athletes on crutches park their cars in the handicap spots.

So to get a parking spot, I had to get to campus very early. Since the engineering building had no library,

I had nowhere to go that early. I would sit in my car and study with the car running and the heater on. In the winter it was cold, but the choice was to come later and not get a parking spot and miss class. I saw very few handicap students on campus and none in the engineering building, so the number of handicap parking spaces should have been adequate, if athletes were not using them.

The Handicap Program was run by the wife of Michigan's governor. I don't know if it was a political appointment or because she had no power, but simple things were hard to get done for handicapped students. For example, the snow and parking made using my wheelchair impossible, so I had to walk to class from my car using my crutches. A dangerous journey on snow and ice, where I realized one slip would be a disastrous fall. So, I took small baby steps, which made the walk slow in the cold of winter.

Once in my classroom, I needed a chair with arms in order to be able to sit and stand. At the start of the semester I arranged for an armchair to be put in my classrooms.

On the second day of class the chair had been removed. I complained to the Office of Handicap Services, but nothing was done. So I would get to class extra early, scour the building for a useable chair, and ask a passing student to move it to my classroom. After several days of doing this, I went to a university vice president's open office hours. He was shocked that his Big Ten University couldn't get a chair put in a classroom. Whatever or whomever he contacted made things happen quickly; the chair was in my classroom and remained there for the rest of the semester.

To compete with the younger students was a matter of hard work. I would spend long hours in the library and labs. It was not unusual for me to be at the university working on a lab project late at night. I made sure I was prepared for tests; all homework was done on time. Being much older than the other students, I didn't make friends or have time to go to sporting events or other student activities. Still I enjoyed the time at the university. The intellectual challenge and being out of the hospital and free to move about made it a joy.

With my studies and my physical therapy appointments, two years at the university went by just as fast as my two years at the community college. I now had my diploma and I was ready to find a job. The university had a job placement program, where students could register for interviews with different companies. So I signed up for several job interviews.

My first interview was with the National Security Agency (NSA). I had the academic credentials they were looking for, but at the end of the interview I knew they were not interested in hiring me. Next was General Motors. The interviewer was looking for a hands-on engineer to work on automotive brakes. I couldn't physically do the job, and that ended that interview. Next was Ford. The interviewer was looking for a robotics engineer. As an electrician, I had experience working on robots, and I had taken classes in robotics in preparation for my Electrical Engineering Degree. However, in the end I didn't get that job either.

So, instead of being disheartened, I returned to the university to get my Master's and improve my resume in hopes of being more employable. Since my grades were good, I was accepted into the Electrical Engineering Master's Program.

That summer an internship was offered to me by the U.S. Navy. It fit with my goal to be more employable by gaining work experience. It was a summer internship program for handicapped students, sponsored by the Department of Defense. The internship was in Washington, D.C., and although it didn't pay much, it was engineering experience and a chance to live independently.

So I was off to D.C. for the summer. I would live in a Gallaudet University dormitory with about twenty other handicapped summer interns. The good news was that I would have my own room, but the bathroom was common to four rooms. Gallaudet University is a university for deaf students. All of the interns could hear, so we were outsiders, and Gallaudet students had nothing to do with us.

I was expected to be independent in the Department of Defense Program: There was no help getting my meals, doing grocery shopping, doing my laundry, or helping me dress. For the first time in a long time I was on my own and I did what was needed to live.

My job in Bethesda, Maryland, working for the Navy was interesting. I worked on acoustics for submarines.

Since I didn't have a classified clearance, my work was limited to detailing the acoustic signature of different systems and trying to make them quieter. The summer went by fast. My weekday routine was to get up early, so I would have the extra time I needed to dress. Then drive from Gallaudet's campus to Bethesda, Maryland, for work. After work return to the dorm, cook and eat dinner, and get ready for the next day by laying out my clothes before getting some sleep. Weekends I wandered around D.C. going to museums and historical places.

One of the places I visited was a hologram museum. It presented the history of holograms and how they are made. I talked to the owner, a man who was trying to develop a film made of holograms. It was an interesting and memorable day, and it ended with me buying a hologram even though my budget was very limited.

On the way to work one day, my car died on the freeway. On the D.C. Beltway, tow trucks cruise continuously to prevent traffic jams from stalled cars or accidents. I didn't have to wait long. A tow truck pulled up, and the driver looked under the hood and determined he couldn't fix the car. He towed the car, with me inside it, to a repair shop where the mechanics found a dead fuel pump. I called into work, explaining why I wouldn't be there that day. It was fixed in a few hours, but the money I earned for that summer was used up fixing the car.

I gained confidence by living independently and working, so it was a very good summer.

I returned to graduate school, competing mainly with foreign students. The university had just instituted a program to recruit very bright foreign graduate students in hopes of gaining a reputation for graduating excellent engineering students. Just as I had in undergraduate school, I out-worked the other students and got good grades. And the year flew by with more late nights studying and work in the computer labs. I was halfway to my Master's degree.

Chapter XVIII
DC Again

One day at the end of my first year of graduate school, I received a phone call. The man introduced himself as Assistant Secretary of Defense and said he wanted me to come to work for him that summer at the Pentagon. He had seen my resume and felt I would be a good fit to work in his office. I was very impressed that a man of this stature would personally call me and so I couldn't say no. Later I found out that there are a lot of assistants to the Secretary of Defense and though he was important, his title wasn't as unique as I had originally thought.

After the call from the Pentagon I got another call. This one was from Edwards Air Force Base in California. They had seen my resume from the Department of Defense's Handicap Program. They also had been impressed with my resume and offered me a full-time position. I explained that I still was in graduate school, wanted to finish my degree, and was not interested at that time. I thought that ended the matter, but I underestimated Darcy, the person on the other end of the phone.

So in a few weeks, I was off to DC again to spend the next summer, living at Gallaudet University's dorm and working at the Pentagon. My work at the Pentagon was reviewing and clearing out a backlog of reports for a department called Live Fire Testing. It was that department's job to test various Defense Department vehicles for survivability in combat. Not exciting work, reading reports all day, but being in the Pentagon and wandering the halls seeing all the history of the place made up for the less-than inspiring task I did every day.

Arriving at the Pentagon, the first thing I noticed was how huge the parking lot was and how many additional small parking lots there were along my arrival route. This indicated to me the large number of employees working there. Even so, I was unprepared for how many people worked in that unique building, and I also was surprised at how big it is. I found a handicap parking spot close to the entrance. As I approached the entrance that I was told to report to on my first day, I noticed the guards. They were professional, and they were no-nonsense, but very helpful. I wasn't used to the security people or systems. Picture IDs were required to get in, and metal detectors were everywhere. This was long before 9/11/2001. The guards called my office and told them I was there. A person from Live Fire Testing came down to meet me. She got me past the guards and showed me the way to the office.

There are no stairs in the Pentagon. Between floors are wide long ramps. I was told that it was designed that way during World War II to move masses of people efficiently and quickly.

In the Pentagon's center courtyard was the "Ground Zero Café," so named because it was thought to be the targeting point for Russian nuclear missiles. I expected it to be an elegant restaurant. Instead, it was a sandwich shop, but it was very popular during lunch hour. And I can say I had a burger at Ground Zero Café (along with thousands of other people).

On top of the walls of the center courtyard were ceramic owls staring down on the cafe. The story behind them is that the Pentagon staff had tried everything to get rid of the pigeons that were infesting the courtyard. They a hired contractor to shoot and poison the pigeons, but nothing worked. Then one day some farmer came up with the idea that pigeons were afraid of owls, so the ceramic owls were bought and placed on the walls. The pigeon problem was solved.

I had a small desk in a small office with two military officers. One of them, a colonel, took his daily stack of mail and threw it in the wastepaper basket without opening a single letter. After several days of watching his routine, I got the nerve to ask him why he threw his mail away.

He said, "If the mail is important enough, they will call me." The practice of throwing mail away continued throughout the summer, and the number of incoming phone calls were few. I learned that military personnel who work in the Pentagon are not permanent employees. They rotate in and out. So by the time someone figured out that the colonel was throwing away his mail, he would be gone.

The dress code required that I wear a suit. So before I left for my summer job, I bought a suit. I had the buttons on the suit coat replaced with Velcro, since my fingers still didn't work. My pants came with buttons for suspenders, so I bought suspenders and attached them to my pants, which kept them up. It was impossible to adjust my pants when I stood up, so the suspenders kept my pants from falling down, which would have been embarrassing to moon people at the Pentagon. My tie was a clip-on because I lacked the finger dexterity to tie a knot. The dress shirt was buttoned ahead of time and pulled over my head. Now I was ready to be a Pentagon government employee.

The suit gave me the opportunity to go to the shops within the Pentagon for the dry cleaners. At the Metro station entrance (the Pentagon has its own train stop) there are shops. They include the dry cleaners, eateries and various other little places. Once a week I would take my laundry to the dry cleaners and stop for lunch. The trip to the dry cleaners gave me an opportunity to wander the halls and use the ramps. I would always walk next to the wall, so if I was bumped or slipped, I could lean against the wall and not fall.

I marveled at the number of people, who were working there and they seemed to be always moving with a purpose, never standing and gossiping. The hallways had exhibits of historical things done at the various offices in the Pentagon. For instance, the Marine Corps office had a display of Iwo Jima. There were also explanations and maps showing the locations of many the offices so a visitor could figure out how to get to the right place. Since the building was a pentagon, its layout of offices was much different than a rectangular building. For instance, an ordinary building's offices have a floor number and a room number. The Pentagon offices have a floor number, section number, and a room number.

One day I was summoned to a huge office. Most of the offices I had seen were small, but this one had a large conference table made of cherry wood in the center of the room and a big desk sitting at the end of the room. The walls were lined with books. Everything was done in cherry wood, and I knew immediately that the occupant of this office was someone important.

A secretary led me into the room and announced my name. A man came from behind the desk, thanked the secretary, introduced himself, and shook my hand. He said he had been the lead civilian at Edwards Air Force Base before coming to the Pentagon. Then he said he had received a call from Darcy at Edwards Air Force Base, the same

Darcy who had called me at the beginning of the summer. She was the woman, who had told me that Edwards Air Force Base was offering me a permanent job as an engineer, the job that I had declined.

My host spent half an hour explaining why Edwards would be a great place to work, and he highly recommended that I reconsider my decision about the job offer. He walked me to the door, and I told him that I would reconsider the job offer.

Although I would not see him again, he had impressed me and I began reconsidering the job offer. At the time it was a difficult decision. Should I continue my master's degree program in hopes of getting a good job, or take this offer and enter the work force as an entry-level engineer? Although the government engineering positions pay less than the private sector, it was a serious job offer. The events of the summer would make it an easy choice.

I returned to my office and the reading of reports. Reports were stacked high, because it was a boring job and no one else in the office wanted to do it. By the end of the summer I had reviewed all the files and made a summary with comments on each report, which the Assistant Secretary of Defense used to make his decisions. At the end of the summer I got a very nice thank you letter and a recommendation from him.

The hours at the Pentagon were long. Even the interns were expected to work more than eight hours a day. I would get back to Gallaudet's dorms late, after all of the other summer interns who worked standard eight-hour days. By the time I got to campus, all the other interns had eaten and gone out for the night. So, I was alone to make dinner and eat. Then prepare my clothes for the next workday, and go to bed.

To get to the community kitchen, I had to walk through the TV room. One night while in the community kitchen, I noticed a beautiful blonde in a wheelchair watching Jeopardy on TV.

It took a few days but I got up enough nerve and tried to talk to her, but she informed me that she didn't talk during Jeopardy. I went back to the kitchen, cooked and finished my meal. By the time I returned to the TV room, she was gone. I would later find out that she was returning to her room after Jeopardy, the only TV show she watched, to study for the upcoming school year. She, like me, was determined to have the work experience and good grades to be employable.

After several failed attempts to catch her before she left the TV room, I skipped my dinner and waited in the TV room for Jeopardy to end, blocked her way out of the TV room, and asked her if she would like to go to dinner with me. She accepted the invitation, thinking we were going to McDonalds, because no one made much money as a summer intern. Little did I know it was the start of a magical summer.

Chapter XIX

Magical Summer

Our first date was to be a dinner at the Kennedy Center's cafeteria. I had planned a late dinner and then up to the roof of the Kennedy Center, which has a spectacular view of the monuments at night. But when we arrived at the cafeteria, it was closed for repairs. Being disappointed, we headed back to the elevator, where we met some Kennedy Center employees. They told us about another restaurant in the Kennedy Center and encouraged us to go to it.

When we got there the maître d' was trying to discourage us from being seated. It was getting late, too late to find another restaurant. Besides, two people in wheelchairs at the Kennedy Center; it would be against their principles not to seat us. So we couldn't be refused. Reluctantly she seated us.

As we sat down, I noticed that the few patrons who were there on a weekday were in formal attire. We were in jeans. However, we soon started talking, and any discomfort about how we were dressed was forgotten, and the night flew by. The waiters and busboys seemed to enjoy the maître d's discomfort with us.

At the end of the meal, Donna said it was time to go back to the Gallaudet dorm rather than do any sightseeing. I was disheartened; I thought she had had a bad time. I was completely unaware how late it was. Time seemed to stand still during that dinner. Donna said it was late, and we both had to get up early to go to work. I looked at my watch, realized, how late it actually was, and my thoughts that I had somehow ruined the evening vanished. Before we left, I asked her for a second date.

The next weekend, for our second date, we went to the Washington Monument together. There was a long line of people waiting to get in and climb the stairs to the top. We started to leave, but we were told by people in the line that being handicapped, meant we could go to the front of the line and ride the elevator to the top. So, we went to the front of the line and waited in a much shorter line to get on the elevator.

As we rode the elevator to the top, the man operating the elevator stopped at each floor and in between floors and opened the doors to show us the historical placards on the walls. He mentioned that we needed to be careful with the doors open for safety reasons that normally because of the construction, the elevator doors are not opened between floors. I think my date's beauty was the reason he opened the doors, when he shouldn't have. At the top we had a great view of the Reflecting Pool, Potomac River, and most of the monuments. Again the day flew by; we rolled around the mall, ate at concession stands, talked and way too soon it was time to go back to the dorm. And I was looking forward to another weekend with her.

Weekends became times for us to explore the Washington D.C. area together. Although neither of us made much money that summer, we used my car to explore. But mostly we enjoyed each other's company.

One such weekend was spent in Annapolis, Maryland. Once our nation's capital, it had a lot of history. Many little shops and inaccessible cobblestone streets, but the history, food and company made it great. The seafood restaurants in Maryland were the best. Driving around we found this little seafood place. The food was cheap, but very good. Fresh Blue Shell Crabs was their specialty and we returned as often we could.

The Smithsonian museums were on our list of places to see. We would visit all of the different museums. It would take a full day to see each museum. Handicap parking was free, so it was a fun, cheap day. Our favorite was the Smithsonian National Air and Space Museum. That was strange because we both would end up working at Edwards Air Force Base, watching the space shuttle land and once a year Chuck Yeager come and break the sound barrier in commemoration of his being the first person to break the sound barrier, which happened at Edwards. The Bell-X1, which Yeager flew to break the sound barrier for the first time, was on display at the Smithsonian National Air and Space Museum.

Another day was spent at the National Zoo. We saw the baby Panda at the zoo. But we spent more time talking about our futures than watching the animals.

We liked the weekend we spent at Williamsburg. Its historically accurate colonial area shops and employees dressed in Revolutionary-period clothing made it a fun day with much to talk about. Donna showed a little of her personality there. We were on top a small hill. There was no short path down, so she, in her wheelchair, went flying down the hill to the sidewalk below. Her long blonde hair flying out behind her, she made it without flipping over. I took the long path around. She visited some of the shops during the time it took me to join her at the village.

We both felt that the summer went by too fast. At the end of the summer of our internship, I drove Donna to the airport for her return to Arizona. We were separated at check-in because without a ticket I was not allowed into the boarding area. We said our goodbyes and promised that we would stay in touch.

She boarded the plane and was gone. I had a long, lonely drive back to Michigan.

Chapter XX
The Beginning of Working

When I got back home, Donna and I stayed in touch by phone. This made me miss her more. I called Edwards Air Force Base about the job offer. I figured Edwards AFB was eight hours from Donna, my home was two days away by car. Plus, the job offers met my end goal to get an engineering job.

The Personnel Department responded to my phone call by flying me out to California for three different interviews. Darcy, who had arranged the interviews, invited me to dinner after the interviews with her boyfriend, Lee. I found it interesting that Lee was like me – a quadriplegic. Lee also worked at Edwards AFB, he was a statistician. He had several insights into working with a disability at a government facility. I hadn't realized the government was exempt for the ADA laws. So, not all the facilities were accessible.

Darcy was a little person and a human dynamo. After meeting her I could see why she didn't take my no for an answer. She was part of the Handicap Program at Edwards Air Force Base, so she had a unique perspective when reviewing resumes and work records of people like me. She was aware of the need for diversity on our military bases, and she was convinced that I'd fit the bill for a number of reasons: Besides being handicapped, I had good grades from a respected engineering program at a major university, had work experience and I was a veteran.

So I wasn't just someone to fill a quota. I could do the job, and my military experience made me a good person to deal with military pilots. Darcy and Lee became our friends for the next twenty years, until Lee's death. Darcy and I still keep in touch.

I received three job offers from different programs at Edwards. I accepted one of them, and started work after a few months that it took the Human Resources Department to process the paperwork. I had more than enough time to fly back home, get my affairs in order in Michigan, say goodbyes and drive my Ford Tempo with its hand controls to the high desert of Southern California. The university professors tried to change my mind. I was the only American in the Electrical Engineering graduate program. They pointed out the lower pay I would receive. But in the end Donna outweighed all their arguments. The three-day drive was an adventure. I took the southern route. With my car loaded with all my possessions, I drove eight to ten hours each day only stopping for gas and food. It took me a whole day to drive across Texas. I stopped and visited Donna on my way through Tucson.

Donna, who by then was finishing school in Arizona, joined me at Edwards Air Force Base for the next summer, where she worked as an intern. She impressed them with her job skills and work ethic. After the summer she returned to Arizona to finish her college degree. The following summer she graduated, was hired as a full-time financial officer, and joined me at Edwards Air Force Base, where we married and started our careers and life together.

Donna would work her way up the financial division. In addition to her normal duties, they gave her a small budget to begin making Edwards AFB handicap accessible. She was part of a program that put the General in charge of the base in a wheelchair for one day. It opened his eyes as to the difficulty of opening doors and getting up curbs. In the end she was an important part of the financial division.

In the Tucson night sky, the North Star shines brightly and helps lost travelers. It reminds me of my wife. We have a joke that between the two of us, we make one whole person. It is hard to imagine life without her. The twenty-six years of marriage has passed too quickly.

One night while transferring into bed, my wheelchair moved. I fell to the floor. While lying there, unable to get to a phone. Donna came up to me and asked me if I was in pain. She then called for an ambulance, let the paramedics into the house. She followed the ambulance to the hospital. She waited through the doctor exams and X-rays to take me home. Although it took all night she never complained or left my side.

One day she went into a pet store for dog food. She came out with dog food and a rescue dog. She has a big heart.

We are different personalities. Donna is outgoing and social. I am introverted and avoid crowds. She is one of those people, you instantly like. So, while working on the Air Force base, she made lots of friends. In contrast I stayed in my cubicle and met very few people. As a result, I became known as "Donna's husband" by most of the base. When I moved to Tucson and began working for the Air National Guard, the first person I met, looked at me and said, "you're Donna's husband." Five hundred miles away .... She had worked with Donna in California. Now that we are retired, she is heavily involved in the community. She is well known and liked. I am the guy, who tags along with her.

If I had a chance to change my life and avoid being wheelchair bound, she would be the one reason, I wouldn't change a thing.

Chapter XXI
The Return to Working

My first assignment at Edwards Air Force Base was in an anechoic chamber. Anechoic means "no echo". It was used to do radar testing. It was a huge hanger that had radar absorbing material on the floor, walls and ceiling. The result the radar would not bounce off the walls and ceiling, but would act similar to a radar outside. Thus allowing a radar test indoors. It would save the cost of flight testing, plus could exactly repeat test points that would be difficult to repeat exactly in the air. The aircraft being tested would bring their engineers and design the tests. So, I would just need to learn the facility and monitor how the facility worked during the test. I fit in well with the staff at the chamber. Being older, when given a task, I would study the task, learn how to accomplish it, independently. Then work to get it done before the test started. I soon was valued for my engineering skills and my handicap became unnoticed by my coworkers. I was just an engineer that could be depended upon to get the job done.

One of my coworkers fit the stereotype of a government worker. He was hired about the same time as me. He would come to work in the morning, go to his desk and stay there all day. He ate his lunch at his desk. After a year someone noticed he didn't have an assignment. He had never been assigned a job and never asked for anything to do. A new aircraft was just starting testing and were desperate for engineers. He was sent there. A few months later he was sent back, because he failed to do the job assigned to him. It was sad because he was intelligent and capable, but he was afraid to fail and that fear prevented him from trying to accomplish anything.

Being an observer of the tests was not enough for me. I would sit in the control room and watch engineers monitor the systems on the airplane. They would stop the test and ask for test points to be repeated, as they worked to understand what was going wrong with their systems. I wanted to do more during the tests, to look at the data, to understand what happened.... So, I transferred to a test organization that tested fighter aircraft.

I enjoyed my time at the anechoic chamber, except for two incidents. At Edwards Air Base because it is surrounded by flat dry lake beds, the wind was very strong. One day while walking to my car, a gust of wind knocked me over on the cement of the parking lot. I had a badly fractured leg that required surgery and a metal plate was inserted in my leg. This was the beginning of the process that stopped me from walking. The second was the government is exempt from the Disability Act. The government doesn't have to make work areas accessible. So, during tests, I had to rely on coworkers to open and close a heavy metal door to gain access to the control room. Also during fire and earthquake drills the elevator was turned off. I had to go from the second floor, which would have been the third floor in a normal building, to the ground floor and out into the parking lot. The staircase went down about ten/fifteen feet to a landing, then turned and another set of steps went down another ten/fifteen feet to the ground floor. The supervisor had the facility buy a "chair" to get me down the stairs. I called it a "suicide chair." It was two poles with canvas between them and small wheels. Someone would have to lower me down, a step at a time. However, the person would be bent way over and trying to lower a two hundred plus pound man down each step, while he was trying to go down the steps. The result would have been, me flying down the steps out of control and smashing into the wall at the bottom of the steps. So, I demonstrated I could get myself down the steps by sitting on the steps and lowering myself a step at a time. It took time, but I was able to go down the steps. I didn't mind the first time, but I felt to do it every drill as wrong. But management didn't see it that way any I continued to do the drills. Also management never replaced the "suicide chairs", despite my explanation of how dangerous they were. To management the "suicide chairs" checked a safety box on some form. So, it really didn't matter how dangerous the chairs were, they looked good on paper.

Chapter XXII

When is a Viper Really a Falcon?

Most of the flight tests in my area were designed by engineers, when I first started in the F-16 test organization. The F-16 is a fighter aircraft, that is fast and maneuverable. The engineering designed tests were straight and level flights that bored the test pilots. So, I engaged with the pilots to design flight tests that tested function in all places in the flight envelope of the F-16. The pilots liked flying at the edges of the envelope, it allowed them to do "fun" maneuvers. As I worked with the pilots, they helped me understand their requirements of how the F-16 should perform in combat. As I gained their trust and respect, my knowledge and tests I designed improved.

One of the pilots I became friends with was Bernie. Bernie wasn't his real name, but it was his "call sign". A name used on radio communication and the name other pilots referred to each other by. Bernie got his call sign by his first day at Edwards AFB. It was tradition that a new pilot go to all the homes of the test pilots in his squadron and have a drink. Having just arrived at Edwards, he was tired and not being big in stature, he couldn't drink the amount of alcohol that visiting all the pilots would require. He passed out part way through the night. The other pilots did not want to spoil the tradition, so they threw him over their shoulders and carried him to the next pilot's house and sat him in a chair passed out until they had their drinks. This continued until the last pilot was visited. So, he got the call sign "Bernie" because he was like Bernie in the movie *Weekend at Bernie's*.

Bernie liked being involved in designing the tests and flying a fighter like a sports car not a bus. So one of the tests for a Radar Warning Receiver (RWR) involved doing an Immelmann, then a Split S maneuvers. The RWR tells the pilot in combat, where the threats to shoot them down are. So, it is important to the pilot that the symbols on the RWR are accurate in combat situations. An Immelmann is an ascending climb with a half loop, then a half roll. The result is flying in the opposite direction at a higher altitude. The Split S is the reverse. The pilot goes inverted (upside down), dives and at the bottom rolls out. The results are flying in the opposite direction at a lower altitude. So flying these two maneuvers together, resulted in testing the RWR in simulated combat conditions. We would do this in military air space, no commercial aircraft were in the same airspace. We would block out the area so there were no other military planes around. Also we would start at 15,000ft altitude, climb to 20,000ft and end up at 10,000ft. It was very safe. We drove out into the desert to be in communication with the aircraft during the testing. Bernie flew the Immelmann and Split S back-to-back flawlessly. At the end of testing we radioed Bernie, telling him the test was complete and good job. Since we were in the middle of nowhere with no people around, we asked Bernie for a flyby. He asked for our position and said "OK". All the engineers from the test were standing around in the desert looking for the aircraft, when we heard the roar of an approaching aircraft. We looked toward the sound and there was Bernie flying toward us at several hundred miles per hour about 100 feet above the ground. When he arrived above us, we expected him to just fly on past. Instead, he hit the afterburners, began a ninety degree climb straight above us. At maybe 1,000 feet in altitude he began to corkscrew as he climbed. Before he was out of sight he leveled out and departed at great speed. The roar from the afterburners was deafening. I think it took a week to get the smile off my face.

The F-16 was nicknamed "Falcon" by the U.S. Air Force, when it was first commissioned. However, anyone who works with the aircraft calls it the "Viper". No one liked the Air Force's nickname, so pilots named it after the fighter on Battle Star Galactica. The name stuck. Officially the F-16 is called the "Falcon", but anyone, who works with it, calls it the "Viper". Funny how the government loses sight of the humanity in its work. To change the designation from Falcon to Viper is such a minor thing, but never will happen.

When I first started with the RWR group within the F-16 test organization, I noticed the test reports had lots of numbers, but little was written as to what the numbers meant. Good for an engineer, but meaningless to the pilot, who has to fly the plane into combat. I contacted Lee for help. Lee was a quadriplegic from a dune buggy accident. Lee also was a mathematician with test experience. He was gracious enough to spend several days training me on test statistics. In the end our group began to report the data in a meaningful way. An added bonus was Uban. Uban was Lee's service dog. Normally you are not to pet them while they are in service. But Lee allowed me to pet and talk to Uban. I think Lee knew that I was an engineer and that I related better to Uban than to people.

There was this story told at Lee's funeral. One of Lee's coworkers knew the rules, but he liked Uban. So the coworker would craw out of his office on the floor to Lee's office door, so as not to be seen by Lee. He then would try to entice Uban to come to him for a treat. Uban, true to his training, ignored him. This brought a lot of laughs and lightened up the funeral.

Chapter XXIII

The End, No Really I'm Done

I spent the next twenty years working at Edwards AFB with a great group of engineers and pilots. Donna became very ill and we needed to move from California to Arizona for better care for Donna. I was lucky to be transferred to a small engineering group that although they worked for Edwards AFB, they were physically located in Arizona.

After five years in Arizona I reluctantly retired. The work in Arizona was fun and challenging. In retirement I sent an email to a test pilot I had worked with, he was just given an important promotion. I congratulated him on his promotion. He took the time to reply. He remembered me as a good engineer, not an engineer in a wheelchair. It seems I have been able to change the perception of me from a man in a wheelchair to a competent engineer over the course of my working for the government. Between being a parent/grandparent, the Marine Corps and being a test engineer my life has had value and meaning, the wheelchair has just been an inconvenience along the way.

Epilogue

My sisters, Diane and Linda, began to write notes from the moment they arrived at the hospital on Day One.

They recorded everything that was said and done. Diane's husband, Dale, is a former naval officer who was accustomed to keeping a careful log on the Bridge of his ship at sea. As a result of his urging, my family members "stood their watch" as a no-nonsense professional naval officer would. Notes not only were detailed; they were made in black ink, on the same kind of paper, with the precise date and exact time of virtually every notation. This book was written partially on the basis of the four hundred pages of notes we saved from the first four months of my Intensive Care Unit experience.

Made in the USA
Middletown, DE
30 September 2018